365 Days of Healthy Eating from the American Dietetic Association

365 Days of Healthy Eating from the American Dietetic Association

Roberta Larson Duyff
MS, RD, FADA, CFCS

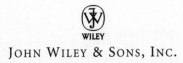

WILEY

JOHN WILEY & SONS, INC.

Published by John Wiley & Sons, Inc., Hoboken, New Jersey
Published simultaneously in Canada

Design and production by Navta Associates, Inc.

For general information about our other products and services, please contact our Customer Care Department within the United States at (800) 762-2974, outside the United States at (317) 572-3993 or fax (317) 572-4002.

Wiley also publishes its books in a variety of electronic formats. Some content that appears in print may not be available in electronic books. For more information about Wiley products, visit our web site at www.wiley.com.

ISBN 0-471-44221-6

Printed in the United States of America

10 9 8 7 6 5 4 3 2 1

Contents

Foreword   vii

Introduction   1

365 Days of Healthy Eating

January   5

February   27

March   46

April   67

May   86

June   108

July   129

August   148

September   170

October   191

November   213

December   233

Foreword

The mystery of eating healthy without sacrificing flavor and favorite foods baffles many people, but with this book as your guide it won't slow your journey toward better health any longer. *365 Days of Healthy Eating from the American Dietetic Association* reveals the secrets to eating well and eating healthy—and many more.

Roberta Duyff's mission has long been to break down the voluminous and sometimes contradictory nutrition information that clutters our cognitive capacity into sensible, positive, and practical advice. It's wonderful to see her put her award-winning skills to work again in a book that offers both help and inspiration for making healthy lifestyle choices every day of the year. The American Dietetic Association commends Roberta on this latest blend of sound science and welcome advice.

On behalf of the members of the American Dietetic Association, may this year's worth of simple steps take you many miles down the path toward better health!

Marianne Smith Edge, MS, RD, LD, FADA
President, 2003–2004
American Dietetic Association

365 Days of Healthy Eating from the American Dietetic Association

Introduction

If every individual could have the right amount of
nourishment and exercise, not too little and not too much,
we would have found the safest way to health.
—HIPPOCRATES

New idea? Not really. This positive, individualized, sensible approach to wellness has been around for nearly 2,500 years—since long before research backed it up. Today's science shows that variety, balance, and moderation in healthful eating and active living are still your best way to feel and look your best, to have energy for all you want to do, and to live a longer, healthier, more productive life.

That's what this day book is about: *you!* It's filled with easy, often fun, can-do ways to eat smart, move more in your daily life, and get the benefits now and later.

Each day offers a few positive, simple-to-do-solutions for daily eating and active living dilemmas—to help you be "well" equipped for daily life. Doing just one tip a day (or a week) will add up and make a difference over the course of 365 (or 366) days.

Scattered through these 366 days, you'll find plenty of how-tos:

 How to . . . Follow a Smart Eating Mind-set

 How to . . . Get Everyday Benefits from Food Choices

 How to . . . Prevent, Delay, or Deal with Health Issues

 How to . . . Buy Right-for-You Foods and Supplements

How to . . . Prepare Food for Good Nutrition, Health—and Great Taste

 How to . . . Get More from Eating

 How to . . . Move More

And you'll find more than sixty recipes for easy, flavorful, good-for-you meal ideas and snacks. I've tested and tasted them all—and they are terrific!

Enjoy seasonal advice day-by-day, or read whatever day catches your attention. At year end, you can start over again. Positive, individualized, sensible, this practical approach is meant for you.

My special thanks to:

Christina Ferroli, PhD, RD; Alice Henneman, MS, RD; Sharon Piano, MS, RD, CFCS; Vicki Walker, MPH, RD; and *Megan Wolfe,* MS, RD, CDN, for carefully reviewing the book for the most up-to-date science, and Sharon Denny and Wendy Marcason, registered dietitians at ADA, for their scientific guidance.

Laura Brown, American Dietetic Association acquisitions editor, for guiding this day book through the editorial process, and *Diana Faulhaber,* ADA publisher, for her support.

Lisa Considine and *John Simko,* John Wiley & Sons editors, for turning these can-do strategies for wellness into a pleasurable book.

Many professional colleagues who generously shared information and flavorful and healthful recipes with an array of ingredients!

Phil Duyff, my husband, colleague, and best supporter, for making wellness a family priority 365 days of the year.

Roberta Larson Duyff, MS, RD, FADA, CFCS

Author note: For in-depth discussion of topics in this book, refer to the comprehensive *American Dietetic Association Complete Food and Nutrition Guide* by Roberta Larson Duyff from John Wiley & Sons, Inc.

About the Author

Roberta Larson Duyff, MS, RD, FADA, CFCS, is nationally recognized as a food and nutrition expert; children's, trade book, and textbook author; consultant; and speaker, who enjoys sharing practical, science-based advice for healthful eating and for the "tastes of good health" with consumers of all ages.

A highly respected author and advocate of "positive nutrition," Roberta's books include the award-wining *American Dietetic Association Complete Food and Nutrition Guide*, *Monthly Nutrition Companion*, *Food Folklore: Truths and Myths Behind the Foods We Eat* (John Wiley & Sons, Inc.), as well as *Nutrition and Wellness* (Glencoe/McGraw-Hill) for teens and *50 Ways to Lower Your Fat & Cholesterol* with Tufts University School of Nutrition.

Her positive and practical consumer advice and healthful recipes appear nationally in popular media, including *USA Today*, *Allure*, *Better Homes and Gardens*, *Cooking Light*, *Ladies' Home Journal*, *Living Fit*, and *Self*, and on nationally broadcast TV, and radio and Web cast appearances. Roberta is a contributing editor to *Today's Health & Wellness* magazine, writes regularly for food-focused Web sites, and is a weekly columnist for the St. Louis *Post Dispatch*.

Passionate about food and its links to nutrition, wellness, and culture, Roberta has served as national chair of the Food & Culinary Professionals of the ADA and as a national leader and member in the Society for Nutrition Education, Consumer Trends Forum International, American Association of Family and Consumer Sciences, International Association of Culinary Professionals, and Les Dames D'Escoffier.

With a passion for ethnic food as a means to cultural understanding and good nutrition, Roberta travels and speaks internationally . . . always in search of flavorful ways to eat for health!

365 Days of Healthy Eating

January 1   📛 Skip Resolutions, Make Plans!

Ever make New Year's resolutions with enthusiasm, only to break them after a few days? For a better chance of success, make *plans*—not just resolutions—for fitness, healthier eating, weight loss, or whatever's important for you.

Here's how:

- *Break your big goals* (resolutions) *into smaller, more specific goals.*
- *List realistic changes that match your goals.*

Specific Goals	Realistic Changes
Walk 30 minutes each day.	Walk 15 minutes during my lunch break.
Eat more vegetables.	Eat salad with dinner.
Lose two pounds in January.	Skip second helpings.

- *Be patient.* Small steps add up over time.
- *Stick with it.* If you waver from your plan, dump any guilt or feelings of failure. Start again where you left off. That's okay!
- *Take another look.* Evaluate your progress every week or two. Update and change your plan if you need to.
- *Reward yourself*—with a new CD or recreation activity, for example, not more food.

Take time today to think about your fit future. What's your . . .

- *Big goal:* _____
- *Specific goals:* _____
- *Realistic changes that may work for you; read through the book each day for ideas:* _____

January 2   Get F.I.T.

Do you realize that a physically active lifestyle helps you get a deeper, more restful sleep? Gives you strength and stamina to do what matters most to you? Gives you some calorie leeway to enjoy another bite? May even extend your life?

With the holiday season over, now's a great time to see if your approach to active living passes the F.I.T. test and offers real benefits! Consider this:

- F-*requency.* Within reason, the more often you do it, the greater the benefit.
- I-*ntensity.* For cardiovascular fitness, fit in time for physical activity that gets your heart pumping. Check with your physician first if you haven't been physically active for a while or if you have a health problem.
- T-*ime.* At least sixty minutes of moderate activity daily is a smart goal. Break it up into shorter segments if you need to.

January 3   The Cold (and Sniffles) Truth

Got the sniffles? Runny nose got you down? Too stuffed up to breathe easily or to taste a great meal? You likely have a common cold—too common during frosty winter days! That said, can any foods, nutrients, or supplements prevent it, or at least minimize your symptoms?

So far, dietary cure-all claims aren't backed by strong scientific evidence. Large doses of vitamin C won't prevent a cold, but its antihistamine effect may ease your breathing. Zinc and echinacea supplements may reduce symptoms, but they also may *suppress,* not improve, immunity. And lobelia, an herbal supplement, may cause harm, from breathing problems and rapid heartbeat to coma, even death!

To relieve cold's symptoms and hasten your recovery:

- *Take time to rest.* Stay away from others if you can.
- *Drink plenty of fluids,* including vitamin C–rich juice (even hot chicken soup). Fluids and warmth help loosen nasal mucous.

January 4   Weighing In on Dieting

Does January mark your renewed goal for a healthy weight? Great! For long-term success and good health along the way, take weight loss slow, steady, smart. A realistic, healthful goal? Most experts agree: ½ to 1 pound of weight loss per week.

To quickly judge a popular diet, check for these ill-fated qualities: promises of quick weight loss, little or no physical activity, rigid meal plans, odd amounts of food, or special food combinations. Diets with these qualities are often boring, dispiriting, even unhealthy. They probably won't work for long and may do harm.

Instead of "dieting," concentrate on smart eating and active living.

- *Watch your portions.* If they're oversized, eat less. (See January 31.)
- *Eat more fruits, vegetables, and whole-grain foods.* They tend to have fewer calories, yet plenty of nutrients. Eat fewer high-calorie, low-nutrient foods (such as soft drinks, candy, salad dressings, high-fat spreads).
- *Go easy on snacks.* Pay attention to how much, how often, and how many snack calories by reading food labels.
- *Move more.* Do something physically active today, even if it's just for fifteen minutes. Gradually increase your activity.

January 5   Peanut Lover?

Love peanuts? Then eat up. Dr. George Washington Carver (today's his birthday) discovered more than 300 ways to use peanuts!

A member of the dried bean family, not a tree nut, peanuts provide protein. And they're also packed with heart-healthy substances—

among them *folate, magnesium, good (monounsaturated) fats,* and two plant substances called *resveratrol* and *plant sterols*—yet no cholesterol!

Enjoy chopped peanuts in salads, on cereal, in baked goods, in smoothies. For a new way to enjoy peanuts, try this:

Peanut-Crusted Chicken

1 tablespoon flour
1 teaspoon seasoned salt
½ teaspoon garlic powder
¼ teaspoon dried tarragon
¼ cup prepared mustard
2 tablespoons honey

1 cup finely chopped, unsalted dry-roasted peanuts
4 boneless, skinless chicken breasts
2 tablespoons butter or vegetable oil

In a pan or shallow bowl, combine flour, seasoned salt, garlic powder, and tarragon; mix well. In a second pan, combine mustard and honey. Place peanuts in a third pan. Dip each chicken breast in flour mixture, then honey mustard, and finally in peanuts to coat. Heat butter in a 10- to 12-inch skillet; add chicken and cook over medium-low heat until internal temperature reaches 170°F and golden brown, 4 to 5 minutes per side. Makes 4 servings.
Source: National Peanut Board

January 6   Supplements—S-age Advice

You don't need to buy out the supplement shelf. But you do need to take the right vitamin or mineral supplement for your age and unique health needs. Remember, food first! Then *if* you need a supplement, here's what health experts advise as a daily guideline, depending on your age:

- *20s, 30s, or 40s: folic acid* (400 micrograms for women) if you're pregnant or capable of pregnancy, to avoid birth defects; perhaps calcium (up to about 1,000 milligrams, more—1,200 milligrams—for menopausal women) and perhaps *iron* (no more than 18 milligrams) if you're a woman with heavy menstrual flow.
- *50s: calcium* (up to 1,200 milligrams for women and men) to protect against bone loss; and *vitamin D* (400 International Units, or I.U.). Vitamin D recommendations go up with age. Women: Stop any iron supplement now.
- *60s: calcium* as noted for the 50s; *vitamin D* as noted for the 50s; and *vitamin B_{12}* (up to 2.4 micrograms) to counteract possible changes in vitamin B_{12} absorption.

- *70s: calcium* as noted for the 50s; *vitamin D* (up to 600 I.U. or less if you drink milk); and *vitamin B₁₂,* as noted for the 50s.

To be supplement savvy:

- *Check the Supplement Facts on any you take* so you don't overdo. A supplement with 100% Daily Value for these or any other nutrients is enough, unless your doctor gives different advice.
- *Make a personal note* to ask your doctor about the right supplements for you. *Note:* Supplements may interact with any medication that you take.

January 7 Cook Savvy—Fat-Trimming Countdown

Ready to reduce your long-term risks for heart disease, cancer, and diabetes? Trimming fat from your food is a great step toward meeting that healthy-eating goal. Health experts advise *20 to 35 percent of calories from fat* (44 to 78 fat grams for a 2,000-calorie daily eating plan). And keep saturated fat (including trans fatty acids) as low as possible.

When you cook today, try a "fat trimmer."

- *Pick flavorful oil.* A little extra virgin olive, sesame, walnut, or herb-infused oil goes a long way.
- *Thicken creamy soup or stew with puréed, cooked root veggies,* such as potatoes, sweet potatoes, parsnips, or turnips.
- *Buy nonstick pans*—to sauté or stir-fry with less fat.
- *Oven bake "fried chicken."* Coat chicken with yogurt, then roll in whole-wheat bread crumbs and herbs. Spray lightly with vegetable oil spray. Oven bake at 350°F in a nonstick pan.
- *Grill or broil, roast or bake, boil or stir-fry*—all low-fat ways to cook!
- *Use a cheese with "character."* Just a little Romano, blue, or Parmesan cheese delivers lots of flavor.
- *Go halfsies.* Toss less butter, margarine, or oil with veggies, pasta, or rice. Ladle less dressing on salad.
- *Follow the ⅔–⅓ guideline: ⅔ of the plate with* veggies, fruits, and grain foods. Fill the rest of the plate with meat, poultry, fish, or cheese.

January 8   The Eyes Have It

An old wives' tale proves true: carrots *do* help you see better.

It has long been known that carrots' beta carotene (which forms vitamin A) helps your eyes adjust to dim light. Cutting-edge research suggests that other antioxidants in plant-based foods may help protect your eyesight from cataracts and age-related macular degeneration.

- Eating foods rich in *antioxidant vitamins* (beta carotene, vitamins C and E) may lower your risk for cataracts, a clouding of the eye's lens.
- *Lutein and zeaxanthin,* found in the retina's macula, protect your eyes from sunlight and other environmental damage. Increase these carotenoids in your eyes by eating plenty of lutein- and zeaxanthin-rich foods.

Choose eye-catching foods to enjoy, starting today.

- *For beta carotene:* yellow-orange fruits and vegetables, including carrots; dark-green vegetables
- *For lutein:* green-leafy vegetables, kiwifruit, eggs
- *For zeaxanthin:* citrus fruit, corn, green vegetables, winter squash, eggs
- *For vitamin C:* citrus fruit, berries, broccoli, brussels sprouts, cantaloupe, green pepper, papaya, tomato
- *For vitamin E:* almonds, corn oil, eggs, peanuts, spinach, sunflower seeds

January 9   Ready—or Not?

Do you want to be and stay healthy? Want sound information to help you do the right thing? Good news: you're in the driver's seat!

Are you ready for healthful eating and active living? Check the statements that sound most like you:

☐ *I want to eat better and move more, but not now.* Okay, but the sooner, the better for your health.

☐ *I think about smarter eating and being active, but don't know what to do.* Great mind-set! Keep a diary to pinpoint what you need to change. Perhaps review it with a registered dietitian.

☐ *I want to make permanent changes for smarter eating and active living.* For good health, make changes you enjoy and can sustain. Can you name one?

☐ *I feel successful only if I totally overhaul my eating and lifestyle.* Think again; even little steps add up and make a difference. Take one small step today.

☐ *I know it's best to make change slowly, step by step.* For most people, gradual change is more sustainable. For weight loss, a half pound per week usually succeeds best.

January 10   Fit for Cold Weather

Cold weather is no excuse to skip fitness routines and nestle in by the TV. A shift of seasons simply gives you different options.

In any weather, the same guideline applies: get 60 minutes of moderate activity every day if you can. In cold weather, try these outdoor activities:

- *Winter sports:* cross-country or downhill skiing, skating, snowshoeing
- *Active leisure:* winter nature walks, snow hiking, sledding
- *Outdoor chores:* snow shoveling, chopping firewood, dog walking
- *Too cold or windy?* Go mall walking inside!

For safety's sake in cold, wintry weather, keep this in mind:

- *Cover up to stay warm.* Your head, hands, and other exposed skin need to be covered. An uncovered head gives off a lot of body heat.
- *Layer your clothing.* Several lightweight layers may keep you warmer than one or two heavier layers.
- *Stay dry.* Moisture conducts cold air toward your skin and heat away. Wicking fabrics help you stay dry as you exercise in winter.

- *Stay hydrated.* Although it may be cold outside, you still can sweat! Bring a water bottle.

January 11   Say OK to Oats

What's for breakfast on this cold, winter morning? How about instant oatmeal, crunchy oat cereal, or an oat bran muffin? No matter how you eat them, oats offer benefits beyond their hearty taste.

A good source of soluble fiber, oats are well known for their heart-healthy benefits, which include lowering blood cholesterol. What's more, the plant substances in oats may help control blood pressure, even body weight (since oatmeal helps you feel full longer). How much helps with cholesterol reduction? Three grams of soluble fiber a day from *all* your foods. One serving of these oat-based foods puts you one-third there: 1 cup ready-to-eat oat cereal, ½ cup cooked oatmeal, or ⅓ cup cooked oat bran. Add oatmeal to muffins, burgers, meatloaf, or stuffing, too.

Try this breakfast treat during National Oatmeal Month:

Peach Muesli with Berries

2 cups oats, uncooked
2 cups coarsely chopped peeled fresh or thawed frozen peaches
1½ cups apple juice
8 ounces vanilla or peach nonfat yogurt
½ teaspoon vanilla
1 cup fresh or thawed frozen blue-berries or raspberries

In a large bowl, combine all ingredients except berries; mix well. Cover and refrigerate for 8 hours or overnight. Serve muesli cold topped with berries. May be stored, covered, in refrigerator for up to four days. Makes 4 servings (1 cup plus ¼ cup berries).
Source: Quaker Oats

January 12   Hunger Strikes? Snack Smart

Will you (or did you) enjoy a snack today? Fine, if you snack smart. Snack for the health of it.

- *Snack when you're really hungry,* not just when you're bored or stressed.

- *Snack with your whole day's food intake in mind,* not just as an add-on. Smaller meal portions allow room for snacks.
- *Choose smart, handy snacks.* Tuck whole fruit or a bag of pretzels in a briefcase or backpack to enjoy when real hunger strikes.
- *Take a sensible portion from the package.* Then put the rest away to put the brakes on mindless nibbling.
- *Read the food label first.* Low-fat snacks may not be low in calories.
- *Snack smart by* not *eating mindlessly in front of the TV.*

Save money and eat smart by packing a handy, healthful snack before leaving home.

- *Your signature snack mix:* any combination of pretzels, nuts, whole-grain cereal, dried fruits
- *Whole fruit:* apple, banana, tangerine
- *Single-serve foods:* canned fruit, applesauce or pudding cup

January 13 Valued Customer

Shopping for value? Value isn't necessarily "supersized" or how much your food dollar buys. True value is the quality and health benefits that your food and drink choices impart.

For the best value for your food dollar:

- *Buy canned or dried beans.* Beans are an inexpensive protein food, loaded with fiber and other phytonutrients.
- *Fill your cart with veggies and fruit.* Fresh, canned, or frozen— nutrition is virtually the same, so shop for the best price.
- *Grow herbs.* It's cheaper and more convenient than buying them.
- *Buy whole-grain foods.* They have more nutrients and fiber than their processed counterparts, for about the same cost.
- *Pack your lunch bag.* You'll save money, and often have more nutrient-rich options than you might have with fast-food eating.
- *Stock your desk with bottled water.* It's cheaper than a vending machine soft drink.
- *Reach for single-serving flavored (perhaps low-fat) milk*—a nutrient-packed snack drink.

And consider this: Down the line, the cost benefits of healthful eating extend to cost savings in your lifelong, personal health care.

January 14 🖋 The "Write" Way to Eat Smart

A bite here, a nibble there, a sip here, another taste there. How much did you eat today?

Want to get a better picture of your day-to-day eating habits? Keep a food diary. It's easier to spot a problem and control temptation, and you have a better chance of reaching your wellness goals and perhaps managing your weight.

Keep records for at least a week or two. Here's how:

- *Pick a system.* A simple notebook or a daily diary works for handwritten records. Or find an electronic tracking system.
- *Track the "5 Ws and H."* Note with whom, what, where, when, why, and how much you eat and drink. Be realistic with amounts.
- *Write down little tastes:* butter on your toast, sugar and milk in your tea.
- *Remember snacks.* That includes vending machine soda, doughnuts, and biscotti.
- *Record any eating "triggers."* Note your mood or hunger level.
- *Give it careful review.* What have you learned about you?

January 15 🌾 Easy as 1, 2, 3, 4, 5

Life's hectic! How can you be assured of eating enough food and variety for good nutrition, but not too much?

Truth is, there's no single way to eat for health. Even your own family members enjoy different foods and flavors, prepared in different ways, and they have different nutrient and energy needs. No matter what your individual style or tastes, there's still an easy, flexible guide for planning a healthful day's worth of meals and snacks for everyone, ages two years or more.

To eat for health:

- *Choose food for variety* among and within the five food groups. Variety is nutritious and tastes good, too!
- *Balance.* Follow food-group serving guidelines to "up" your chances of eating the right amount of nutrients and calories (energy) for your age, gender, and activity level. If your portions are bigger or smaller than food-group servings, that's okay—*if* the day's total adds up to *your* whole day's serving advice.
- *Make calories count.* Pick mostly foods that deliver more nutrients. Go easy on foods high in fat and added sugars.

How Many Food-Group Servings?

Food Group	Children ages 2 to 6, most women, some older adults *(about 1,600 calories)**	Older children, teen girls, active women, most men *(about 2,200 calories)**	Teen boys, active men *(about 2,800 calories)**
Bread, cereal, rice, pasta (especially whole-grain)	6	9	11
Vegetable	3	4	5
Fruit	2	3	4
Milk, yogurt, cheese (preferably fat-free or low-fat)	2 to 3**	2 to 3**	2 to 3**
Meat, poultry, fish, beans, eggs (preferably lean or low-fat)	2 (total 5 ounces)	2 (total 6 ounces)	3 (total 7 ounces)
Fats, oils, sweets	Eat sparingly	Eat sparingly	Eat sparingly

* Calorie levels if you choose low-fat, lean foods and if you use fats, oils, and sweets sparingly.

** Older children and teenagers (ages 9 to 18 years) and adults over age 50 years need 3 servings daily. During pregnancy and lactation, the milk-group recommendation is the same as for nonpregnant women.

January 16   Eye on Size

How much is a food-group serving? It's not necessarily a helping, a plateful, a small garnish, or the entire contents of one food package. It is a specific, standardized amount of food, meant to help you judge your own portions and estimate how much you eat.

Your portion may measure as more or less than one food-group serving; for example, a one-cup portion of cooked pasta is really two bread-group servings.

The size of your portion doesn't matter. What does matter is whether your portions add up to the day's recommendation (or a several-day average), without overdoing.

Learn visual guides. Either measure your food, or use these cues to become a good judge of your portions.

How Much Is a Food-Group Serving?

Food Group	One Serving, About the Size of . . .
Bread	1 slice bread, 1 pancake, or 1 waffle = a stack of three computer diskettes 1 cup dry cereal = a baseball ½ cup cooked pasta or rice = a small computer mouse
Vegetable	1 cup raw leafy vegetables = a baseball ½ cup cooked vegetables = a small computer mouse 10 French fries = a deck of cards 1 small potato = a small computer mouse
Fruit	½ cup sliced fruit = a small computer mouse 1 medium fruit = a baseball ¾ cup juice = a 6-ounce can ¼ cup raisins = a large egg
Dairy	8-ounce glass of milk = a small (8-ounce) milk carton 8-ounce yogurt = a baseball 1½ ounces hard cheese (Cheddar) = two 9-volt batteries or a C battery
Meat and Beans	2 to 3 ounces meat, poultry, or fish = a deck of cards or a cassette tape One ounce meat equals: • 2 tablespoons peanut butter = a roll of film or a Ping-Pong ball • ½ cup beans = a small computer mouse or a deck of cards

January 17 🜨 Cho-LESS-terol

Do you know your vital signs for heart health: your cholesterol levels and your blood pressure? For total cholesterol level, normal is less than 200 mg/dL (milligrams per deciliter). The higher your level, the greater your risks for heart attack or stroke. So, even if your cholesterol level is borderline high (200 to 239 mg/dL), work toward a lower, heart-healthier goal.

Four key strategies can put you in the *total* "cholesterol countdown": (1) if you smoke, stop; (2) eat smart; (3) move more; (4) lose weight if you need to. Make your eating style low in saturated fat and cholesterol, moderate in fat overall, with plenty of fruits, veggies, and whole-grain foods. If that's not enough, you might need cholesterol-lowering medication, too.

Know your HDL- (good) cholesterol, LDL- (bad) cholesterol, and triglyceride levels, too. Even with normal total cholesterol, your LDLs could be too high, and your HDLs, too low for heart health. Normal is: HDLs, 60 mg/dL or more; LDLs, less than 200 mg/dL; triglycerides, less than 150 mg/dL.

Start today; eat to help bring blood cholesterol levels within a healthy range.

- *Go for five.* Have five to nine daily servings of fruits and vegetables (seven for physically active women, nine for physically active men).
- *Enjoy beans (legumes).* One or two bean meals a week gives variety.
- *Eat six to eleven grain products* (at least three whole-grain) servings daily.
- *Eat fish, poultry without skin, and lean cuts of meat.* Cook them in low-fat ways.
- *Eat mostly fat-free and low-fat dairy foods:* two to three servings daily.

January 18 🛒 All Dried Up

Need an easy way to get your "five to nine a day" for fruits and vegetables? Reach for dried fruit. There's lots more than raisins, dried apricots, and dried plums (prunes) on store shelves today.

Are dried fruits as nutritious as fresh? Overall, yes, except the drying process destroys a hefty amount of vitamin C (no problem if it comes from other fruit or juice). Some dried foods, such as raisins, provide more iron, too. Why? Drying concentrates minerals, as well as sugars and calories. Dried fruits tend to have plenty of fiber, too.

Sensitive to sulfites? Look for sulfite-free dried fruit.

Try "dried"—and remember that one serving is just ¼ cup.

- *Mix up a dried snack "to go."* Mix any dried fruit with nuts, pretzels, and perhaps popcorn.
- *Sweeten with dried berries.* Top salad, cooked rice, yogurt, or cereal with dried berries of all kinds.
- *Batter up.* Add dried fruits to bread or cookie dough, or pancake, waffle, or muffin batter.

January 19   Passport to Health—Eating Chinese Style

Gung Hay Fat Choy! Happy Lunar New Year! Whether you eat out or in, enjoy Asian flavors and foods today, and get their good-for-you benefits.

Traditional Chinese meals have plenty of vegetables, rice, and noodles (that's their benefit), yet they're modest with meat, poultry, and fish. Besides their vitamins and minerals, vegetables in Chinese dishes are loaded with antioxidants, fiber, and other healthful phytonutrients, or plant substances.

If you eat out, go easy on higher-fat dishes: *fried* versions of egg rolls, wontons, dim sum, noodles, rice, fish; *breaded* sweet-and-sour dishes. Some soy sauces and dips are high in sodium. If you have high blood pressure, ask for low-sodium sauce.

Cooking today? "Wok" your way to health. Rather than deep-fry, go for stir-fry (cooked in very little oil), mixing any ingredients you enjoy!

- *Start chopping lots of different veggies:* asparagus, bok choy, broccoli, carrots, green and red peppers, mushrooms, snow peas, spinach, sprouts—all cut in bite-size pieces.

- *Add Asian flavor* with chopped garlic, ginger, lemongrass, scallions, hot peppers.
- *Prepare modest amounts of protein foods.* Use beef, chicken, pork, seafood, or firm tofu, cut in ½-inch pieces. Let vegetables outweigh protein foods two or three to one.
- *Heat the wok (or skillet) with 1 tablespoon of oil.* When it sizzles, start cooking: first the meat and herbs, then add veggies. Cook just until the vegetables are tender-crisp.
- *Serve* over brown or white rice, or Chinese noodles.

January 20   Soup-er Bowl

Super Bowl Sunday is just around the corner. Why not make it a *soup-er* bowl by cooking a hearty soup, chock-full of great-tasting, good-for-you ingredients?

Celebrate National Soup Month.

- *Double up for more flavor and nutrition.* Experiment. Combine two hearty convenience soups (canned or frozen) to create your own recipe, perhaps chunky minestrone plus beef barley soup. Find convenience soups with less sodium.
- *Serve in a bread bowl.* Hollow out individual round loaves (try whole-wheat). Fill with chunky vegetable soup or your family's favorite chili.
- *Make it heartier.* Add frozen or canned legumes (beans, peas, lentils) and other veggies to convenience soups to step up the flavor, visual appeal—and the vitamins, minerals, fiber, and other phytonutrients, too.
- *Get creamy with milk.* Prepare condensed cream soups with milk (perhaps evaporated fat-free milk), not water. Any way, milk's calcium-rich!
- *Garnish for flavor and more.* Use shredded cheese for more bone-building calcium, seasoned almond slivers for extra vitamin E, chopped sun-dried tomato for a bit of beta carotene and lycopene.
- *Take it up a notch.* Spark up the taste with no-salt flavorings: hot sauce on corn chowder or chopped cilantro on tomato soup.

January 21 🍎 Orange You Glad!

Slice into a tangy grapefruit. Peel a tangerine. Squeeze lemon in your tea. Citrus fruit, now in its peak season, offers you an ample supply of good nutrition!

For most people, oranges mean *vitamin C.* But did you know that citrus also supplies an ample amount of *folate, potassium,* and *dietary fiber* (soluble), all potentially heart-protective, among their other functions?

Beyond that, citrus fruits brim with health-promoting plant substances: *flavonoids* with heart-healthy and anticancer qualities, *limonoids* that may inhibit tumors, and *carotenoids* with their antioxidant activity, of which some may protect your vision.

Add sliced citrus to your salad, or squeeze citrus into a belly-warming hot drink like this one:

Orange Cider

3 cups orange juice
1 cup apple juice
1 2-inch piece stick cinnamon

¼ teaspoon whole cloves
1 orange, sliced (optional)

In a saucepan combine orange juice, apple juice, cinnamon, and cloves. Bring to boiling; reduce heat. Cover and simmer for 10 minutes. Strain to remove cinnamon and cloves. Serve warm. If desired, float orange slices on top. Makes 4 servings.

Source: Florida Department of Citrus

January 22 🚶 Mind Over Matter

At any age, most Americans aren't active enough—although they may think they are! In fact, only about 26 percent get enough exercise; about 46 percent come up short; and about 28 percent are inactive. Studies show that adults tend to overestimate how active they really are. Do you?

What's the downside of inactive living? The link to overweight and obesity, heart disease, diabetes, some cancers, osteoporosis, back pain, to name a few. What's the upside of moving more? Good health, perhaps a longer life—and a better quality of life overall!

Commit to an active mind-set to help you move more.

- *Treat your exercise routine like any important appointment.* Don't break it!
- *Get in touch with your reality.* Log real time (in a notebook or a PDA) spent on moderate activity to know how active you really are.
- *Take 10.* Get your 60 minutes of active living daily in 10-minute segments, if that's easier for you.

January 23   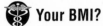 Your BMI?

Do you know your BMI (Body Mass Index)? Do you know what your number means?

BMI is meant to *screen for,* not diagnose, overweight or obesity. It's a tool to evaluate your weight in relation to your height. A higher-than-healthy number (above 25) suggests a higher risk for weight-related health problems such as heart disease, hypertension, stroke, diabetes, some cancers, arthritis, and breathing problems.

Although BMI is a good health indicator, it's not the last word. With less muscle but more body fat, a person's BMI still may fit the healthy range (18.5 to 25); conversely healthy, muscular people might have a BMI above 25. What counts is your overall health. Diagnosing a weight problem and determining your healthy weight is best determined with your physician.

Learn more about your "number."

- *Check your BMI online.* Go to Partnership for Healthy Weight Management (www.consumer.gov/weightloss/bmi.htm) or National Heart, Lung, and Blood Institute (www.nhlbisupport .com/bmi/bmicalc.htm).
- *Find out more about what your BMI means.* Contact a registered dietitian, or ask your health care provider to help you.

January 24   No "Nos," No "Shoulds," No "Nevers"

Ever hear your inner voice say: "You *should* order a salad," or "No fried food!" Chances are, these mental commands are hard to stick to, at least for the long term. And they take pleasure away from eating to stay fit.

Truth is, healthful is full of positives: a variety of flavorful, eye-appealing food combinations, the good feeling of eating enough without being overstuffed—and the interaction of eating with others.

Smart eaters do this. Do you?

- *Focus on the positives.* Choose grilled vegetables, quick-to-eat fruit, tangy yogurt, hearty whole-grain foods, or fresh, tender seafood. Ultimately that's more motivating!
- *Dump the negatives.* Never say "never eat," and avoid "avoid," "cut out," and "don't." Skip "shoulds" and "have tos," also. These tactics leave you feeling guilty when you "break" the rules—an almost sure bet for failure!
- *Stick to "small bite" advice.* Unless you have an allergy or perhaps another health problem, you can eat a small amount of any food if your overall choices are healthful.

January 25   Certified, But Qualified?

Looking for a personal fitness trainer? With so much interest today in fitness, many people seek a personal trainer to help customize their physical activity regimen.

That said, being certified doesn't mean qualified. No state or federal laws regulate the many certification programs of personal trainers. Some states require a health-related university degree (perhaps in exercise physiology) and an exam; others certify with a few weeks of training. Few trainers are educated to give nutrition guidance. Don't confuse them with physical therapists or registered dietitians.

If you want the services of a personal trainer:

- *Talk to a qualified health professional.* Ask your physician or a registered dietitian (RD) for a referral. For nutrition advice, find a local RD at www.eatright.org.
- *Meet the trainer.* Before you sign up for services, ask about his or her education, experience, and training approach. Is it right for you?

- *Go prepared.* Share your medical history, health status, and any physical limitations.
- *Set goals together.* Make them attainable and safe for you. If your goal is fitness, you don't need to set goals to be an athlete.
- *Ask questions* about the approach, the equipment, the pace, the skills.
- *Follow-through—and enjoy!*

January 26   Eat Your Broccoli

Broccoli, bok choy, brussels sprouts: what do they have in common? They're all cruciferous vegetables that begin with the letter *b*!

Cruciferous vegetables (named for their tiny cross-forming flower petals) belong to the cabbage family. The family portrait includes everything from arugula to watercress—with cauliflower, collards, kale, kohlrabi, mustard greens, radishes, rutabaga, Swiss chard, and turnips in between.

Why so healthful? First their nutrients: *beta carotene* (which forms vitamin A), *vitamin C,* and varying amounts of *calcium, iron,* and *folate.* Second, cruciferous vegetables have a unique phytonutrient array that includes cancer-fighting *indoles* and *isothiocyanates,* and fiber.

Enjoy this three-cruciferous-veggie dish:

Garlicky Greens

1 tablespoon extra-virgin olive oil
¾ cup sliced leek, white part only
½ cup chopped scallions (about 3),
    both green and white parts
1 tablespoon minced garlic (2 large
    cloves)
3 cups chopped kale
3 cups collard greens cut in
    ½-inch ribbons

1 cup chopped broccoli
5 cups fresh spinach
1 cup fat-free, reduced-sodium
    chicken broth
Salt and freshly ground black pep-
    per, to taste

Heat oil in a large, heavy skillet over medium-high heat. Add leek, scallions, and garlic. Sauté until leek is limp, about 4 minutes. Add kale, collards, and broccoli, stirring until wilted. Mix in spinach. Add broth and simmer, stirring occasionally, until greens are tender, about 15 minutes. Season to taste with salt and pepper. Makes 4 servings.

Source: American Institute for Cancer Research

January 27 ✎ What's the Temp?

Do you wash your raw meat, poultry, or fish to remove bacteria that cause food-borne illness? Wrong approach! The only way to kill bacteria in meat, poultry, and seafood is through proper cooking to a safe inside temperature. That includes hamburgers and meatloaf; surface bacteria can get mixed inside ground meat dishes. As you cook, use a meat thermometer to check for doneness.

Not in the habit of using a meat thermometer? Today's a good day to start.

- *Shop for a meat or "instant read" thermometer.*
- *Insert the thermometer in the thickest part* (not by the bone or fat).
- *Check the temp:* 140°F for pre-cooked ham; 145°F for fish; 160°F for pork, medium-cooked beef or lamb, ham (not pre-cooked), ground meat, or egg dishes; 165°F for ground chicken or turkey, or leftovers; 170°F for poultry roast or breast; 180°F for a whole chicken or turkey.

January 28 🍎 Plum Good

Prunes have a new name: dried plums! With it comes new data. Great-tasting dried plums offer more health benefits than just keeping your body regular.

Dried plums score high in *antioxidants,* plant substances that may help protect you from heart disease and some cancers. They're also good sources of *fiber* (soluble and insoluble)—3 grams in five dried plums. They supply minerals: *boron, copper, iron, magnesium, potassium.* And whether dried or fresh, their natural *sorbitol* is key to their laxative effect.

To cut fat from baked goods, substitute an equal amount of puréed plum for at least half the butter, margarine, or oil.

Try this snack dip on sliced apples or whole-wheat crackers:

Curried Dried Plum Dip

1 8-ounce package cream cheese or
   low-fat cream cheese, softened
1½ teaspoons curry powder
½ cup (about 3 ounces) chopped
   dried plums

¼ cup mango or other fruit chutney,
   chopped if needed
¼ cup sliced green onions
2 tablespoons chopped almonds,
   toasted (See March 8.)

In small mixing bowl, beat cream cheese and curry powder until smooth. Fold in remaining ingredients. Serve as a spread for sliced fresh fruits or crackers. Makes 14 servings.

Source: California Dried Plum Board

January 29   Speed Read a Food Label

Pressed for supermarket time? Still want to shop healthy?

Here's how to quickly decipher the Nutrition Facts on food labels, using the "5-20 guide":

- *Nutrient Facts are listed as percentages of Daily Values (DV), in amounts per serving.* For a single nutrient, 20% or more is a lot, and 5% or less is a little.
- *For nutrients you may need less of,* such as fat, saturated fat, cholesterol, and sodium, look for foods with 5% or less DV per serving.
- *For nutrients you may need more of,* such as vitamins A and C, calcium, iron, and fiber, look for foods with 20% or more DV per serving.

A few more quick label-reading tips:

- *Check claims.* If the front of the label gives a clue for "high" or "more," "less" or "free," Nutrition Facts gives the specifics.
- *Remember the rule of doubles.* Eating double the servings means double the DV for any nutrient and for calories.

January 30   Join the 10,000-Step Club

Venture a guess. How many steps do you think you take daily: 500, 1,000, 5,000, more? Some studies suggest that 10,000 steps daily is about right to help with weight management. Stepping that much may take conscious effort!

Who's counting? You!

- *Buy an inexpensive pedometer,* clip it on your belt or waistband, and watch your steps add up.
- *Start with a baseline.* For a week or two, count your total steps, then calculate a daily average.
- *Log in.* Before you hit the pillow, record your day's steps.
- *Put on your sneakers and start moving!* Set a stepped-up goal; perhaps start with your highest day so far.
- *Step up gradually.* Try 500 more steps per day for a week, until you comfortably reach the 10,000-steps-a-day target. Stick with it!

January 31   Too Much of a Food Thing?

Imagine you're scooping a bowl of ice cream, serving a plate of pasta, or making a perfect burger. Are your portions right-sized or super-sized?

Not sure? You're not alone. Research shows many consumers underestimate their portion sizes—and their caloric intake. The causes may in part be cultural. Restaurant supersizing, larger cup holders in new cars, larger dishes and cups—all contribute to our distorted ideas about portions. And our hurry-up society means we may overeat before our body cues say, "I'm full." It takes about twenty minutes for your brain to register you're full.

The portion savvy:

- *Know visual cues.* Read January 16.
- *Compare their own portions to the package label's serving sizes.* For your size portions, figure the calories. Surprised?
- *Eat from a plate, not the package!* That way you'll know how much you really eat.
- *Enjoy "slow food."* Pay attention to your food—the flavors, the surroundings, and the amount you eat.

February 1   Take Heart!

The average heart beats about 100,000 times every day and pumps blood through nearly 60,000 miles of blood vessels to deliver oxygen and nutrients to your body cells.

To commemorate American Heart Month, reduce your chances of heart disease.

- *Eat smart.* Enjoy many different fruits, vegetables, and grain products including whole grains; lean meat, poultry, legumes, fish (at least 6 ounces weekly); and fat-free and low-fat dairy foods.
- *Keep your body weight healthy.* Balance the calories you eat with those you burn. Stay physically active.
- *Keep your blood cholesterol and triglyceride levels normal.* (See January 17.) Limit the saturated fat, cholesterol, and trans fatty acids in what you eat. To keep triglycerides within a healthy range, avoid excess calories from any source, including alcoholic drinks.
- *Keep your blood pressure normal.* To help you do so, keep your weight healthy. Eat foods with less salt, and limit alcoholic drinks.

Do something heart healthy today.

- *Commit to a goal.* Choose from those listed above. Take one small step, one realistic change, toward it today.
- *Make an appointment.* Get your cholesterol level and blood pressure checked if you haven't done so for a while.

February 2   Your "Pearly" Whites

Whatever your age, give your smile some attention.

Eating cheese, yogurt, or milk helps keep teeth healthy. These foods not only contain calcium and phosphorus, which may help remineralize teeth, some cheeses also increase saliva flow, which helps fight cavities.

Oral health (teeth and gums) has benefits beyond appearance and speech. Proper chewing also promotes healthful eating. Keeping your teeth and gums healthy starts when you're young.

During Dental Health Month, take time to improve a dental habit.

- *Brush and floss.* Twice daily, use fluoride toothpaste and a soft toothbrush that reaches everywhere in your mouth. Floss between teeth daily, moving floss up and down, away from your gum, to remove particles and plaque that stick there.
- *Skip sips.* Drink a sugary beverage all at once. Sipping drinks, sucking candies, or nibbling chips bathes your teeth with cavity-promoting sugars for up to 40 minutes after you're done! *Caution:* Supersize drinks extend "sip time."
- *Snack smart.* Limit snacking to reduce exposure to cavity promoters. Any carbohydrate foods—candy, chips, crackers, cookies, or pasta—that stick to and between teeth promote cavities.
- *Make an appointment for a dental checkup and regular cleaning.* Call today!

February 3 Parent for Smart Eating

Do *you* eat your broccoli and carrots, or do you push them to the side of your plate? Do *you* drink milk with a meal, or a soft drink instead? Do *you* mindlessly nibble while you watch TV?

Chances are, your child will do what you do—if not now, then probably later. In mimicking you, a child tries grown-up behavior and hopes to please you. Your most powerful parenting technique is being a good role model.

Help your child eat smart!

- *Do what you say.* The next time you order a fast-food drink or eat when you're stressed or bored, think about the messages you send.
- *Give your child and family enough table time.* Rushing through a meal is stressful and doesn't give a child time to learn body signals for fullness. Slow eating helps avoid overeating.
- *Reward with attention, kind words, and hugs,* not with desserts,

candy, or other food. Food rewards such as candy, for your child or you, make them seem better than other foods.

February 4 🍎 One Potato, Two Potatoes

Did you know that potatoes come in many different colors: red, blue, purple, and yellow? And nearly everyone loves them! Celebrate America's favorite vegetable during National Potato Lovers' Month.

It's well worth celebrating. For 100 calories, one medium 5-ounce potato (skin on, plain, not fried) provides: 45% Daily Value (DV) for *vitamin C,* an antioxidant that protects against cell damage; 21% DV for *potassium,* which helps reduce the risk of high blood pressure; and 12% DV for *fiber,* protective against some cancers and perhaps heart disease. What's more, potatoes contain *glutathione,* an antioxidant that may help protect against cancer.

The challenge? We eat many of those potatoes as high-fat fries and chips! Nurture the potato lovers in your family in a lower-fat way by oven-roasting sliced potatoes tossed in olive oil.

As a snack or appetizer, try lower-fat potato tapas.

Potato Tapas

1   pound Russet potatoes, thinly sliced
1   tablespoon vegetable oil
2   tablespoons finely chopped onion
Salt to taste
½ cup diced tomatoes

2   tablespoons seeded, diced Anaheim chilies
1   cup shredded low-fat Cheddar cheese
1   cup prepared salsa

Preheat oven to 400°F. Spread potato slices evenly on a nonstick or greased cookie sheet. Brush with oil and sprinkle with onion and salt. Bake 25 to 35 minutes, or until potatoes are cooked and browned. Sprinkle tomatoes, chilies, and cheese on top. Bake 5 minutes longer or until cheese melts. Serve with salsa. Makes 6 servings.
Source: Washington State Potato Commission

February 5 Read the Fine Print

Are banana chips, chicken hot dogs, air-popped popcorn, and reduced-fat peanut butter any better for you than their traditional counterparts?

Fact is, banana chips, like potato chips, are fried and high in fat and calories. Unless labeled as "reduced fat," chicken hot dogs have as much fat and calories as those made with pork or beef. Air-popped popcorn still may be drizzled with butter or butter-flavored oil. Even if reduced-fat peanut butter has less fat, it may have more corn syrup and as many calories to compensate.

If you pick up a "healthy-sounding" food today, read the fine print first before you buy.

- *Do a fact check.* Compare the label's Nutrition Facts with those of the traditional version of the food.
- *Turn to the ingredient list.* Look at both versions: traditional and nutrition-positioned foods. Remember, ingredients are listed in order, from most to least.
- *Find the serving size.* Make sure you're comparing the same amounts.

February 6   Cook Savvy—Fiber Up

Fiber is the broom that helps give your intestines a clean sweep. This plant substance multitasks, too. A fiber-rich diet helps protect you from colorectal cancer, heart disease, diabetes, constipation, hemorrhoids, and diverticulosis—and perhaps helps you keep a trimmer waistline.

How much do you need? The daily advice is: men, 30 to 38 grams; women, 21 to 25 grams, depending on age. Kids' needs are figured as age plus 5 (e.g., age 10 + 5 = 15 grams fiber).

When you prepare food, make it a fiber-boosting day.

- *Be a bean counter.* Beans have at least 5 grams fiber per half cup. Add garbanzos to your salad, soybeans to chili, and any variety to veggie soups, stews, or pizza.
- *Enjoy skins.* Edible peels on potatoes, apples, grapes, peaches, and eggplant have more fiber than the insides.
- *Sneak fiber in.* Add bran or oatmeal to meatloaf, or ground flaxseed to batter or dough.
- *Go for whole.* Use whole-grain ingredients: brown rice in stir-fries and pilaf, whole-wheat flour for half the flour in baked goods.

- *Boost veggies.* Add extra veggies to casseroles, pasta dishes, pizza, salads, and sandwiches.
- *Boost fruit, too.* Serve berries or whole fruit (edible skin on) over angel food cake, cereal, pancakes, salad, and yogurt.

February 7 Safety in Motion

Accidents happen! Each year health-promoting intentions of active living lead to serious injuries. The reason? Ignoring safety guidelines. Today get more safety savvy with your physical activities.

- *Sign up for a class.* Learn how to do a new sport safely.
- *Carry identification.* This is especially important if you have a health problem, such as diabetes.
- *Wear the right shoes.* Get shoes meant for your sport, with proper treads and foot support.
- *Wear safety gear.* Wear a helmet if you ride a bike, downhill ski, snowboard, ride a horse, in-line skate, or sled. For in-line skating and snowboarding, wear elbow pads, knee pads, wrist guards, and gloves, too.
- *Wear reflectors* if you run or walk at dusk or after dark; better yet, wait for daylight.
- *Apply sunscreen* if you're active outdoors, even on a cold or cloudy day.

February 8 Great Ways to Graze

Do you eat "three squares" a day, or "graze" with five or six smaller meals? Either way is okay—*if* you control any temptation to overeat.

Eating small, frequent meals (instead of two or three bigger ones) may help keep your energy and blood sugar levels steady. Some studies suggest a slight blood cholesterol–lowering effect when you eat this way. And, if you're well disciplined, grazing can help you maintain a healthy weight by helping you control your appetite: no big hunger surges! The challenge: Planning and calorie control for five or six smaller meals daily may take more effort.

To keep grazing within your control:

- *Stretch.* Keep your total food intake to the daily guideline—just divide it into six meals instead of three. (See January 15 and 16.)
- *Think small.* Enjoy appetizer- or tapa-size portions. Fruits, vegetables, and whole-grain foods are great for small mini-meals that are nutrient-rich yet without too many calories or too much fat.
- *Slow down.* Give your body enough time (at least 20 minutes) to feel satisfied with smaller portions.
- *Pay attention.* Smart grazing is strategic eating. Mindless, often constant, nibbling isn't!

February 9 Do Energy Bars Boost Energy?

If you reach for an energy bar as an afternoon pick-me-up, consider this: You'll likely get a food that's high in calories and perhaps high in fat—without an immediate energy boost. Other foods may offer more health benefits and perhaps better taste!

Energy bars were first launched as a convenient, quick-energy snack for endurance athletes. Unless you need to replenish your energy stores in a workout lasting ninety minutes or more, energy bars offer no special benefit. Even then, a slice of bread or a few crackers are just as good, for less cost and fewer calories.

Is an energy bar good after a casual workout? You may eat more calories than you just burned. If you eat a protein bar to build muscle, foiled again. Only working your muscles can do that.

If you reach for an energy bar anyway:

- *Read the label.* Check the calories and nutrients in a single serving. See if the energy bar *is* just one serving.
- *Fit energy bars into your whole day's smart eating strategy.* That way their calories won't add up to more than you need.

February 10 🌾 Your Think Tank

Ever utter these words: "Where did I leave my keys?" or "I just forgot what I was going to say." Maybe you're tired or stressed—or maybe there's an eating connection.

For your brain to function, it needs fuel. Unlike muscles, your brain doesn't store glucose for energy production. Instead, it constantly draws on glucose in fluid surrounding your brain cells. This glucose comes from regular meals, with carbohydrates (in vegetables, fruits, legumes, and grain foods) as the best fuel source. Beyond that, adequate amounts of several B vitamins, vitamins C and E, iron, and zinc are essential for normal brain function.

Can certain foods promote short-term memory? Healthful eating does that. Other food substances—in blueberries, strawberries, dried plums, fatty fish—are under study for their possible roles in short-term memory. Stay tuned!

Even before research offers more insight, think to eat, and eat to think.

- *Eat smart.* Enjoy blueberries, strawberries, dried plums, and fatty fish, such as salmon. No matter what research ultimately says about their link to memory, they're good for you!
- *Skip the urge to skip meals.* You need to freshen your glucose supply, especially in the morning. Breakfast gives a healthful start to the day.
- *Enough rest and plenty of physical activity helps, too.*

February 11 ✍ Culinary Herbs—Boosting More Than Flavor

Do you use oregano, rosemary, mint, and other aromatic herbs in your cooking? A teaspoon or two may add *scents*—and *sense*—to any dish. Studies show that phytonutrients from just a teaspoon or two may boost the health benefits of your favorite foods.

Like fruits and vegetables, herbs and spices are filled with "phytos" with their possible antioxidant benefits. That means they may help prevent and repair cell damage that could lead to heart disease, cancer, and other health problems.

Research on culinary herbs is new. So far, we know that oregano, marjoram, dill, peppermint, rosemary, and thyme pack some antioxidant punch. Fresh herbs appear to have more antioxidant power than dried.

Marry taste and health in your kitchen.

- *Season with more herbs and less salt* for more benefits, more antioxidants, less sodium, and plenty of flavor.
- *Flavor your veggies and fruit to boost their "phytos."* Experiment with dill on green beans or sweet potatoes, peppermint on carrots or berries, rosemary on fruit or tomatoes, thyme on peas or onions.
- *Toss herbs into any dish.* Try mint or lavender in smoothies or yogurt, basil in tomato salads, and cilantro on eggs or salad greens.
- *Add herbs and spices (nearly calorie-free) instead of extra fat.*

February 12 Can Do, Can You?

Fresh or canned? You might think you could taste the difference in recipes but in taste tests, fruit smoothies, bean burritos, and other popular recipes got high marks for flavor, appearance, aroma, and texture whether they were made from fresh, frozen, or canned ingredients. Nutritionally speaking, studies show, they're about the same, too. Both fresh and canned veggies lose some B vitamins and vitamin C when cooked. The key to nutrition is proper storage, handling, and cooking.

Stock up for canned convenience during National Canned Food Month.

- *For less sodium:* "no-salt-added" vegetables, soups, stews
- *For fruit and vegetable variety:* blueberries, mandarin oranges, mango, papaya, pumpkin, okra, soybeans, different beans (legumes), precut tomatoes, turnip greens, others
- *For omega-3s:* albacore tuna, anchovies, mackerel, salmon, sardines
- *For less added sugar:* fruit in natural juice

- *For less fat:* tuna in spring water
- *For more flavor:* pasta sauces, soups, vegetables, fruit—seasoned with herbs, spices, chilies, or other flavor ingredients

Winter Gazpacho

1 14½-ounce can chicken broth, preferably reduced sodium or Italian seasoned

1 14½-ounce can diced "pasta-ready" tomatoes, undrained

1 8-ounce can zucchini in tomato sauce

2 ounces (about 1 cup) torn day-old Italian or French bread

1 15- to 15½-ounce can chickpeas (garbanzo beans), rinsed and drained

Freshly ground black pepper

In a medium saucepan, bring broth and tomatoes to a boil. Stir in zucchini with sauce and bread. Reduce heat and simmer for 10 to 15 minutes, stirring to mash bread into the soup. Bread will become very soft and will nearly dissolve to thicken the soup. Stir in chickpeas and simmer 1 minute or until heated through. Season to taste with pepper. Makes 4 servings.

Source: Canned Food Alliance

February 13   Kissable?

Is your breath fresh enough for tomorrow's Valentine's Day kiss?

Odors from foods such as onions and garlic are absorbed into the bloodstream, transferred to the lungs, and exhaled. Until they're digested and eliminated, they may cause bad breath. For dieters, infrequent eating may cause it, too. Other causes? Poor dental hygiene, tobacco residue, or a dry mouth.

If you struggle with bad breath:

- *Brush well (twice daily); floss well (daily).*
- *Brush your tongue, too.* Or get an even more efficient tongue cleaner at your local pharmacy.
- *Ease up on onions and garlic.*
- *Nibble the garnish; chew the seeds!* Parsley, mint, anise, and dill or fennel seeds freshen your breath naturally.
- *Drink more,* especially if your mouth is dry. More saliva flow helps oral bacteria wash away.
- *Use a mouthwash as a quick fix.* The effect doesn't last long. And remember, sucking sugary mint candies promotes tooth decay.

- *Stop smoking.* Being more kissable is another good reason to quit!

If bad breath persists, check with your dentist or physician—it may signal a more serious health problem.

February 14   For the Love of Chocolate

Chocolate's romantic symbolism reaches far back to Mayan and Aztec traditions, and to the belief that chocolate contains mysterious properties that seduce the heart. No wonder sending and enjoying chocolate defines today's Valentine's Day celebration!

Enjoying chocolate may seem decadent. Yet growing scientific evidence offers a more balanced view. Two fats in chocolate may be heart healthy: *stearic acid,* which doesn't seem to increase LDL- (bad) cholesterol, and *oleic acid,* a monounsaturated fat that may help raise HDL- (good) cholesterol. Chocolate also contains *flavonoids* (a type of antioxidant) that may be cardio-protective. *Tip:* Dark chocolate has more antioxidants. If you're a chocolate lover, go easy— since chocolatey foods are generally made with high-fat, sugary ingredients.

Does chocolate give an "emotional buzz"? It does contain stimulants—caffeine and theobromine—but not enough for a significant effect. It has small amounts of phenylethylamine, a mild mood elevator—but not enough to be an aphrodisiac. Although substances in chocolate aren't physically addictive, you may learn to crave their pleasant flavor.

To control your chocolate craving:

- *Stretch the pleasure.* Enjoy one or two small chocolates; ration the rest for later.
- *Satisfy your craving with a small-size chocolate bar.*
- *Enjoy a mug of Mexican-style hot chocolate*—made with milk and cinnamon.

February 15 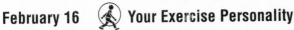 Gone Fishing

Do you eat fish at least twice a week? That's the heart-healthy advice of the American Heart Association. Fish is low-fat and protein-rich. Most of its fat is unsaturated, which is good.

There's more. Fattier fish—albacore tuna, anchovies, mackerel, salmon, lake trout, among others—are rich in omega-3s (a type of unsaturated fat). Eating these fish as part of overall smart eating may help lower your blood cholesterol level and reduce your risk for artery buildup, heart attacks, high blood pressure, and rheumatoid arthritis. They may lower cancer risk, too, but it's too soon to know for sure.

Fish is as easy to prepare as meat or poultry.

- *Pick a lean cooking method.* Grill fatty fish since it won't flake; bake or broil any fish.
- *Flavor simply.* Brush with chutney, olive oil, fruit purée, or prepared sauce. Sprinkle on herbs, chopped sun-dried tomatoes, or roasted garlic. Top with toasted almonds, vegetable or fruit salsa, or a little stir-fried veggies.
- *Cook thoroughly.* For finfish (such as cod, flounder, halibut), 10 minutes at 425°F for every inch of thickness, to an internal temperature of 145°F.

February 16 Your Exercise Personality

Outgoing, reserved, independent, cautious—when it comes to physical activity, which describes you?

- ☐ *Socially active:* likes to work out with a friend or group, needs a push to more move
- ☐ *Independently active:* likes to set a personal workout routine and pace, plans ahead, can't wait to get moving
- ☐ *Creatively active:* prefers spontaneous physical activities instead of a set workout plan, enjoys being active—once started

You may be a combination of all three, but one style likely describes you best. Recognizing your personality may help you plan an active living approach that motivates you most.

Set your movement goals. If you're . . .

- *Socially active:* Sign up for group classes or a team sport, or find a buddy to walk or swim with.
- *Independently active:* Walk or jog a measured course around the neighborhood, swim laps to match your goal, do circuit training, or use exercise equipment with set goals.
- *Creatively active:* Give yourself permission to walk in the snow, ride your bike, golf when a friend calls. Promise yourself you'll do it—nearly everyday.

February 17 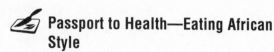 Passport to Health—Eating African Style

Looking for new ways to enjoy vegetables and fruit? Enjoy dishes from the African American culinary tradition. Among the ingredients indigenous to northern and western Africa are okra, yams, watermelon, black-eyed peas (cow peas), and certain greens.

African yams and greens of African origin aren't generally available in the United States. But for four hundred years beta carotene–rich sweet potatoes, kale and collard, mustard, and turnip greens have taken their places here. Groundnuts (peanuts) are also a staple in West African cooking. Add them to soups and stews.

During Black History Month, enjoy nutrient-rich vegetables that blend African American and Southern cuisine.

- *Simmer chopped collard greens* with lean ham, onion, and red pepper flakes. *Tip:* 10 minutes cooking time is enough.
- *Simmer cut-up sweet potatoes* with butternut squash until tender. Drain; mash with only a touch of butter or margarine, salt, and pepper.

Okra and Stewed Tomatoes

1 teaspoon olive oil
½ cup coarsely chopped Spanish onion
1 cup (about ¼ pound) fresh okra, cut into ¾-inch pieces

1 8-ounce or 14-ounce can stewed tomatoes
Freshly ground pepper to taste

In deep saucepan, heat oil over medium-high heat. Sauté onion until it softens, about 4 minutes. Add okra and sauté 3 to 4 minutes, until it turns bright green. Add tomatoes, bring to boil, reduce heat, and simmer until okra is crisp-tender, about 5 minutes. Season to taste with pepper. Serve immediately, so okra doesn't get gummy. Makes 4 servings.
Source: American Institute for Cancer Research

February 18   Slow Down, You're Eating Too Fast

. . . gotta make your mealtime last! "Slow food"—a European movement to eat more slowly and savor the pleasures of the table—is gaining attention in the United States and may offer more benefits than you think.

- *First the obvious.* Slow eating gives you time to savor foods' flavors and to enjoy the company of family or friends around the table.
- *Less obvious.* Slow eating may help with weight control. Since it takes about 20 minutes for your brain to register that your stomach is full, you more likely eat less.

Take time to "hear" your hunger cues.

- *Put down your fork or spoon* between each bite.
- *Eat with chopsticks*—if they slow you down.
- *Pay attention to foods' flavors, aromas, and textures.* Chew thoroughly.
- *Enjoy conversation and social time* around the table. Talk about the food.

February 19   Designer Labels

Breakfast cereals, nutrition bars, sports drinks—more and more foods formulated for women now appear on supermarket shelves. Do you need them? Are they *only* for women?

These products are formulated to fill nutrition gaps. They may have more folate for a healthy pregnancy and a healthy heart, more iron to replace what's lost in menstrual flow, more calcium to protect against menopausal bone loss, soy with isoflavone's hormonelike benefits to relieve the discomforts of menopause. Except that women need more iron, these same foods may benefit men, too.

That said, with too many fortified foods, you may overdo on nutrients, especially if you take a supplement already. Traditional foods can fill in any nutrition gap just as well, and perhaps for less cost.

If you reach for gender-targeted foods:

- *Read the label.* Check the sugar, sodium, and calorie content on the Nutrition Facts. Buy only if they fill a need you don't meet another way.
- *Be realistic about the promise.* Remember, no food offers a magic bullet for health.

February 20   Are You a Bean Counter?

Do you count on beans for their health-promoting benefits?

"Beans" actually refers to the whole legume family: chickpeas (garbanzos), lentils, peanuts, and soybeans—as well as black, kidney, lima, navy, and pinto beans, and many others.

Legumes are well known for their protein and fiber benefits, especially in meatless dishes. Count on them for *phytoestrogens* that may be cancer protective and for *folate,* which protects against birth defects and may be heart-healthy, too. Feel gaseous when you eat beans? See July 27.

Try to enjoy beans at least twice weekly.

Healthy Cajun Beans and Rice

1 tablespoon vegetable oil
½ pound turkey sausage or other low-fat smoked sausage, cut in ½-inch-thick slices
1 medium onion, chopped
1 medium green bell pepper, chopped
2 cloves garlic, minced
6 cups cooked rice
1 15-ounce can kidney beans, drained and rinsed (or 1½ cups cooked dry-packaged kidney beans)
1 15-ounce can navy or Great Northern beans, drained and rinsed (or 1½ cups cooked dry navy or Great Northern beans)
2 14½-ounce cans Cajun-style stewed tomatoes
1 teaspoon dried oregano
½ teaspoon hot pepper sauce
1 cup thinly sliced green onions

Heat oil in a large skillet over medium-high heat until hot. Add sausage, onion, green pepper, and garlic. Cook, stirring, 7 to 10 minutes or until sausage is browned and onion is tender. Add rice, kidney beans, navy beans, tomatoes, oregano, and hot pepper sauce. Cook and stir 2 to 3 minutes more until well blended and thoroughly heated. Sprinkle with green onions, and serve immediately. Makes 12 servings.

Source: American Dry Bean Board

February 21   Too Busy to Eat?

Do you ever get so busy with daily living that it seems easier to skip a meal than take the time to fit one in? The irony is that meal skipping can make you less productive. Studies show that meal skipping often leads to losses in concentration, energy levels, and perhaps problem-solving skills.

Meal skipping is no way to lose weight—although some people think it is. Often it leads to overeating on snacks, or at the next meal, resulting in even more calories consumed and perhaps more pounds gained.

Even if you're rushing today, take time to eat.

- *Stop for a deli sandwich to go.* Ask for tomato slices and other veggies. Order a carton or bottle of milk with it.
- *Pack whole fruit, crackers, and cheese to take along.*
- *Buy ingredients for a speed-scratch meal at home:* precut veggies and skinless chicken strips for a fast stir-fry, or mixed salad greens and deli meat for a quick chef's salad.

February 22   Pick Up Your Pace

Has physical activity become part of your daily life? Terrific! Ready to pick up your pace?

A longer, more intense workout may offer more health benefits—if you're active already (and if your doctor says it's okay). Start gradually: perhaps walk faster or longer, or lift heavier weights.

If you're ready, try this to crank your physical activity up a notch:

- *Alternate your pace.* If you're walking already, alternate. Walk for a minute, then run or walk even faster for a minute, and so on. Same thing works for swimming and cycling.

- *Go the distance.* And make it farther, perhaps extending your walk a mile or two through an interesting neighborhood or pleasant park. Or spend 10 more minutes on the exercise bike or cross trainer.
- *Set a new goal that's realistic for you.* Join a fun run, fun walk, or bike-touring event.

February 23   No Crossovers

Before you blame a flu bug for an upset stomach, consider that food-borne illness often starts at home.

How can you avoid it? Frequent handwashing, proper cooking temperatures, and prompt refrigeration, for starters. Just as important is to keep food safe from *cross contamination.* Always separate raw meat, poultry, and seafood, which may harbor "unfriendly" bacteria, from food that's ready to eat.

How well do you prevent food-borne crossovers? Do you . . .

- *Use one utensil to taste, another to prepare food.*
- *Keep raw meat, poultry, and seafood on your bottom refrigerator shelf* to make sure their juices don't drip onto other foods.
- *Always use separate plates:* one for raw meat, poultry, or seafood, another for cooked foods.
- *Use two cutting boards:* one for raw meat, poultry, and seafood; the other for bread, fruit, vegetables, and other foods that are ready to eat.
- *Before using them again, wash knives and mixing spoons.*
- *Keep clean*—hands, dishcloths, counters.

February 24   Some Like It Hot!

Mild to hot, chili peppers are in high demand—and give food more than flavor. Flavorwise, chiles' hot substance, *capsaicin,* stimulates pain receptors in your mouth. The more capsaicin, the hotter the chile. From mildest to hottest: anaheim pepper, then ancho or poblano peppers, then jalapeño or chipotle peppers, then serrano peppers, and then "hot" habañeros (Scotch bonnets).

As a phytonutrient, capsaicin may have antioxidant—cancer-fighting or heart-protective—action. Their *vitamin C* and *beta carotene* also make chilies healthful, with red chilies having more beta carotene than green ones.

To reduce the "fire" if you cook with chilies:

- *Protect sensitive skin.* Wear rubber gloves, or wash your hands carefully after handling chilies. Never touch your eyes or any sensitive places when you handle hot chilies.
- *Remove the seeds and the inner membranes.* That's where most capsaicin resides.
- *Soak chilies in cold salty water for about 60 minutes.*
- *Go easy.* Add just a little chili pepper at a time.
- *Drink milk or eat yogurt.* The protein in dairy foods binds to and washes capsaicin away.

February 25   Shaking the Salt Habit

Need to watch your salt intake? Are you one of the 39 percent of Americans who have high-normal or high blood pressure? Since high-salt eating is linked to high blood pressure, you're smart to choose and prepare foods with less salt.

But what if you like salty tastes? Then try to retrain your tastebuds. The less salt you eat, the less you'll want. After all, you weren't born loving salty tastes. You learned it, so you can unlearn it, too. Taste before you shake today; a dish may not need more salt.

If food needs a flavor lift:

- *Pep it up with pepper.* Chili peppers or hot pepper sauces come in different degrees of "hot."
- *Add a splash of vinegar.* Herbed, balsamic, wine, or rice vinegar give a flavor spark to sauces, soups, and salads.
- *Use MSG* for flavor with one-third the sodium in the same amount of salt.
- *Shake on a salt-free herbal blend.*

No-Salt Herbal Blend

½ cup dried oregano
½ cup onion powder
2 teaspoons garlic powder
2 teaspoons dried basil
2 teaspoons dried marjoram

2 teaspoons dried rosemary
2 teaspoons dried thyme
¾ teaspoon dried sage
¾ teaspoon black pepper

Blend ingredients. Makes 1 cup.

Source: St. Louis Herb Society

February 26 Eating in the Fast-Food Lane

Do you eat fast food at least once a week? About a third of all consumers do. That's okay sometimes, but many fast foods deliver a lot of calories and fat, yet they often come up short on vitamins, minerals, and fiber.

The next time you head for the "fast-food lane," try one of these seven easy ways to eat smarter:

1. *Downsize.* For fewer calories and perhaps less fat, sugar, or sodium, order regular, not supersize, portions.
2. *Color your sandwich!* Add tomato, lettuce, and peppers to your burgers, subs, and deli sandwiches.
3. *Mind your buns.* Order your sandwich with whole-wheat bread or buns if you can.
4. *Trim the trimmings.* Go easy on creamy spreads, such as mayo, tartar sauce, and special sauce. Go for catsup, mustard, or barbecue sauce instead.
5. *Stay "side" wise:* Split a small order of fries or onion rings. Order a salad (light on dressing) instead; go for slaw or fruit.
6. *Sip smart.* Pick your beverage for better nutrition—milk for a calcium boost, or juice instead of soda.
7. *Look for options:* wraps, stir-fry bowls.

February 27 From the Inside Out

Ever feel that if you could just lose (or gain) a few pounds you would feel content, worthy, and in control? News flash: Body size can't do that. And this "outside-in" approach to dieting instead may set you up for failure. Instead look at yourself from the inside out.

Start today to care for the "you" inside.

- *List five personal joys or successes.* Tell someone about them.
- *Give yourself permission to stop whatever stresses you.* Take control of just one stressful moment at a time. Do it again tomorrow, and the next day, too.
- *Do something small for yourself,* perhaps a 15-minute walk before dinner. Hug yourself for your success.

February 28   Howdy, Partner!

Getting enough iron? If you're female, maybe not! Yet, to feel ener-gized, your body needs enough iron to carry oxygen to body cells where energy is made.

To replace iron lost monthly in menstrual flow, women need more iron than men: 18 milligrams of iron daily for women (ages 19 to 50 years), compared to 8 milligrams for men. (After age 50 or so, women need 8 milligrams of iron daily, too.)

Where do you get iron? Among the best food sources are meat and poultry. Beans, eggs, and whole-grain and iron-enriched cereals, breads, and other grain products supply iron, too, but you'll need to partner them with a vitamin C–rich food or a little meat to maximize their absorption.

To boost iron benefits from food, enjoy:

- *A citrus or a tomato garnish* with quiche, an omelet, or a vegetar-ian dish
- *Chopped ham or smoked turkey* to flavor bean chili, or rice and beans
- *Vitami C–rich fruit or fruit juice* with meatless meals. Try orange slices on a peanut butter sandwich or tomatoes with a rice-bean dish.
- *Strawberries or melon* on your breakfast cereal

February 29   Leap to Health

Run, walk, jump, *leap*—commemorate Leap Year's *bonus day* in action. Consider these 24 hours as "found time" to get active, stay active, or become even more active. Spread it out in 10-minute increments, or do your 60 minutes a day of moderate activity all at once. Either way, you benefit.

Here's how:

- *Trimmer body.* Being active is an effective way to lose weight, or keep extra pounds off.
- *Stronger bones.* You need to walk, run, or do anything that carries your weight.
- *Stronger muscles.* You'll find it easier to lift, move, and carry things.
- *Stress relief, better sleep.* Emotional fatigue is replaced by physical fatigue.
- *More stamina, coordination, and flexibility.* A "feel-good" feeling has health benefits, too.
- *Less risk from health problems.* Heart disease, some cancers, and diabetes are linked to inactivity.
- *Injury protection.* An in-shape body avoids danger, slips, or falls more easily.
- *Better mental outlook.* Being active promotes a "can do" feeling.
- *Feel younger.* Active living helps slow some effects of aging.

Leap forward today. For starters:

- *Park farther away,* then walk with a long stride and quick pace.
- *Take the stairs;* skip any moving sidewalks.
- *Carry your groceries;* leave the cart behind.

March 1   Smart Eating—Just Say "Know"

Are eating healthy and active living important to you? An overwhelming 85 percent of American consumers say it is, according to a recent survey. Hungry for timely nutrition information? Almost 60 percent of consumers say they are.

So where do you go for reliable advice? See a qualified professional: a registered dietitian (RD) with a four-year degree in nutrition, or a dietetic technician, registered (DTR) with a two-year nutrition degree. Both complete nutrition internships and must stay up-to-date with ongoing nutrition education.

This National Nutrition Month, find a reliable expert for science-based advice.

- *Click on to expertise* from the American Dietetic Association at www.eatright.org for updates on nutrition issues and for a referral to an RD near your home.
- *Call your local hospital or university Extension office* for a local nutrition expert.
- *Read what RDs write* in popular media (magazines or newspapers, books, or Web site columns). Look for the RD initials after the author's name.

March 2   Got You?

Have a "gut reaction" (intestinal discomfort) to milk? Thirty million Americans are lactose intolerant. The "dairy" good news: If you're lactose intolerant, you probably still can enjoy milk with your cookies.

Lactose intolerance isn't a milk allergy. Instead the body simply doesn't make enough of the enzyme lactase to digest lactose properly. Lactose sensitivity varies; you may be more or less sensitive than someone else.

How do you know if you're lactose intolerant? See your doctor if you suspect a problem; symptoms could be something else.

To get milk's many nutrients if you're lactose intolerant, try this:

- *Drink milk with food.* Diluting lactose makes it easier to digest.
- *Enjoy less more often.* A ½-cup serving may be easier to digest than a cup.
- *Opt for "whole."* Whole milk with more fat slows digestion so lactose is released gradually.

- *Get "cultured."* Yogurt and buttermilk with active cultures may help digest lactose.
- *Say cheese.* Aged cheeses, such as Cheddar, Colby, and Swiss, may be better tolerated.
- *Reduce lactose.* Buy lactose-reduced milk, or use a lactose-reducing tablet in any milk.

March 3   🍎   Sweet Sweet Potatoes

Have a sweet tooth? Nibble a sweet potato!

Think about this. One-half cup of sweet potatoes delivers more *beta carotene* (antioxidant) than 12 cups of broccoli. Sweet potatoes also supply *vitamin E,* another antioxidant, and *potassium,* too. Raw sweet potatoes make an easy low-calorie, nearly fat-free snack. They deliver *fiber,* even more with the peel on. Sweet potatoes give a no-sugar-added sweetness to a meal, and cooking makes them sweeter yet.

Sometime this week, do this with sweet potatoes:

- *Blend* cooked and chilled sweet potatoes in breakfast smoothies. (Quick tip: Use canned sweet potato purée.)
- *Cut* them in strips for oven-baked fries.
- *Substitute* sweet potatoes for white potatoes or apples in recipes.

Rosemary Roasted Sweet Potatoes

2 pounds sweet potatoes, roughly cut into 1½-inch pieces
3 large cloves garlic, peeled and coarsely chopped
1 tablespoon chopped fresh rosemary
2 tablespoons olive oil
¼ cup toasted pine nuts (See March 8.)
2 tablespoons chopped parsley
1 teaspoon salt
¼ teaspoon coarsely ground black pepper

Preheat oven to 375°F. In roasting pan, combine sweet potatoes, garlic, rosemary, and oil. Toss to blend well. Roast for 50 minutes, turning occasionally. Just before serving, sprinkle with pine nuts and parsley, and season with salt and pepper. Makes 8 (½-cup) servings.
Source: North Carolina Sweet Potato Commission

March 4   🛒 Eat Out, Eat Right

Remember when eating out was a special occasion? That's changed!

On average, today's American consumers eat out more than four times a week and spend more than 46 percent of their food dollars away from home. That said, eating out needs as much smart-eating attention as eating in.

When you eat out, order wisely, savor the food, enjoy the company.

- *Order less:* appetizers as main dishes, no extra sides, one drink, not two.
- *Know where more calories lurk:* creamy sauces; fried foods; high-fat extras, such as margarine, butter, sour cream; salad dressings; sugary desserts.
- *Have it your way.* Ask for sauce on the side, veggies without salt or butter, or grilled rather than fried fish.
- *Outsmart the menu.* Decide what you'll eat when it's served; push the rest aside, or take it home for tomorrow.
- *Enjoy the flavor adventure.* Try a dish with an uncommon veggie or fruit: parsnips, fennel, guava, pepino, and so on.

March 5   🏃 Work in a Workout

Do you work in a daily workout? Too busy? Overloaded family demands and workday? You don't need to make a huge time commitment to make health-promoting moves.

For an everyday active lifestyle:

- *Put physical activity on your calendar.* Schedule it for first thing in the day or before preparing supper. Like brushing your teeth, make active living a habit.
- *Divide it up.* Four 15-minute moves add up to the 60 minutes of moderate activity health experts advise.
- *Make it fun.* Pedal around the neighborhood. Play Frisbee with your kids. Dance! Do some heavy gardening.
- *Think of a missed opportunity or two.* Try walking with friends or

family while you catch up on their news. Can you eat a quick lunch, then walk?

- *Forget the guilt.* If you miss a few days, just start again. It's okay!

March 6   Well "Thaw-t" Out

How do you thaw frozen foods? In the fridge? In the microwave oven? Under running water? Or do you risk food-borne illness by thawing food on your kitchen counter?

Bacteria that cause food-borne illness grow fastest between 40° and 140°F. A single bacterium can multiply to trillions in 24 hours.

Cool is the rule during National Frozen Food Month and all year long. For safety's sake, thaw food:

- *In the fridge at 33° to 40°F,* with a pan underneath so drippings don't contaminate other foods. Thaw on the lowest shelf. Allow time, sometimes 24 hours or more.
- *In the microwave oven* only for foods you'll cook completely right away.
- *Under cold running water* in a clean, sanitized sink. Make sure the water doesn't drip and contaminate other foods. Limit the time to 2 hours or less, and change the water every 30 minutes.
- *As part of cooking* if there's time to cook longer than normal. Stir often. Check the internal temperature with a meat thermometer for thorough cooking.

March 7   Claim Check

Pushing your cart through the grocery store aisles? Will you buy the cereal labeled with "more," the juice with "added," or the bottled water labeled as "fortified"?

Before you slip products into your cart, use these consumer tactics to pick what's right for you:

- *Learn the language.* Know that label terms like "more calcium" or "low-fat" mean what they say. The government regulates the definitions.

- *Get specific.* Use the labels' Nutrition Facts to identify the calories and the nutrients in a serving, and perhaps to compare a few similar products.
- *Stay shopping smart.* If a product has "more" of something (perhaps vitamin D), do you really need the extra? If another has "less" of something else (perhaps fat), are you prudent in your whole approach to eating? As important, was the food or drink healthful to start with, even before it was "more" or "less" modified?

March 8   Feel Like a Nut?

Nuts to you! Just a small handful of nuts is packed with *protein*, other nutrients, *fiber*, and health-protective plant substances. Stick to a small serving so calories don't add up. In fact, 1½ ounces of nuts a day may reduce your chance of heart disease if the sat fats and cholesterol in your food choices are low!

Different nuts have different benefits: almonds for the most *fiber*, almonds and hazelnuts for the most *vitamin E* (an antioxidant), pecans for more cancer-fighting *ellagic acid*, Brazil nuts for more *selenium* (another antioxidant), cashews and pistachios for more *potassium*, walnuts for *omega-3 fatty acids*. Many nuts also have *phytic acid*, which may reduce cancer risk and help control blood sugar, cholesterol, and triglycerides.

Wonder about the fat? It's mostly *monounsaturated*—the kind that doesn't raise your blood cholesterol. And nuts are cholesterol-free, too.

Pick an easy *nut*ritious culinary idea today.

- *Use nuts as a condiment.* Sprinkle on soup, salad, yogurt, chicken or fish, or cooked veggies.
- *Switch nuts* for different benefits. Try chopped hazelnuts in salads, walnuts in pesto, or pistachios on baked fish.
- *Try this crumby idea:* Mix finely chopped nuts in a bread crumb topping.
- *Give a toast to nuts!* Toast nuts in a dry skillet over medium heat for 3 to 5 minutes, shaking often, to intensify their flavor.

March 9 🍴 Confront Emotional Eating

Feeling stressed, angry, or bored? Hungry or not, do you check out the refrigerator or vending machine?

Mood-triggered eating can turn into poor nutrition that leads to excess calories and unwanted weight gain. That may cycle to more negative feelings—perhaps guilt or poor self-esteem.

So stress won't get the best of you:

- *Try positive self-talk.* Forget what's wrong; think of one or two things that feel right. If it helps, talk aloud.
- *Work it off with exercise.* Don your walking shoes and take a brisk walk. Turn on some music and relax muscle tension as you move to the beat.
- *Give yourself permission for a "time-out."* Try a bubble bath, soft music, a relaxing book, or giving a hug to someone who needs it as much as you do.
- *Get professional help if you need it!*

March 10 🌾 Divide and Conquer

When it comes to eating smart, you've probably heard a lot about variety, balance, and moderation. Great, but just what does a healthful meal look like? How much of what foods belong in a meal?

Visualize a healthful meal by dividing your plate into four quarters. (To avoid overeating, picture an 8-inch, not a 10-inch, plate.)

- *Fill three sections with vegetables, fruit, and rice, pasta, bread, or other grain products.* (Make portions reasonable, not overflowing. Choose whole-grain foods as often as you can.)
- *Fill one section with lean meat, poultry, fish, or beans.* (A meat serving is the size of a deck of cards, or 3 ounces.)
- *Add a glass of low-fat milk* (or, if you're a vegan, a calcium-fortified soy beverage).

March 11 🛒 Nutrient Supplements, or Not?

Do any of these describe you? (Check which ones.)

☐ Limited milk intake or sun exposure?

☐ Vegetarian?

☐ Eating problem, or a digestive or a liver problem?

☐ On a very restrictive weight-loss diet?

☐ Unable (or unwilling) to eat in a healthful way?

☐ *(if you're female)* Heavy menstrual flow, able to become pregnant, pregnant or breast-feeding, or menopausal?

If so, a nutrient supplement may be wise. Before you self-prescribe and put yourself at health risk, get supplement savvy!

For an informed decision on supplements:

- *Evaluate your food choices first.* If your meals and snacks supply enough nutrients, you probably don't need a supplement.
- *Check with your doctor* for the right supplement, in the right amount, for the right reasons, for you.
- *Know what you're taking.* Read the label's ingredient list and Supplement Facts.
- *Pick a "multi," not a "mega."* One hundred percent of a nutrient's Daily Value (per dose), in a single or multivitamin/mineral supplement, is probably enough. Anything more can be harmful or at least an unnecessary expense.
- *Stick with a smart dosage.* Don't take more than the label dose per day.
- *Be cautious about combining.* Taking nutrient supplements with medication (over-the-counter or prescription) or herbal supplements may have dangerous side effects. Ask your doctor or pharmacist.
- *Remember, out with the old, in with the new.* Toss any supplement older than the expiration date.

March 12   Getting Any Older?

At least you may not *feel* any older! You can't stop time, but eating smart and moving more may slow the biomarkers, or physical changes, of aging and help you feel younger longer. These biomarkers include:

- *Your muscle mass and strength.* Adults lose about 7 to 8 pounds of muscle a decade.
- *Your body's fat.* With age, body fat replaces muscle. It adds up especially around the midriff, where it's riskier.
- *Your rate of energy use.* For basic work, your body uses about 2 percent less energy for every decade.
- *Your bone density.* Bone loss is part of aging.
- *Your "numbers."* Cholesterol and blood sugar levels often go up with age, increasing, respectively, heart disease and diabetes risks.
- *Your body's thermostat.* A sense of thirst diminishes.
- *Your aerobic capacity.* With age, the body doesn't use oxygen as efficiently.

You can slow these physical changes—even reverse some:

- *Stay physically active.* Regular moderate activity helps keep muscles strong, pumps oxygen to muscles, burns energy faster, and promotes healthy weight and healthy "numbers." If weight-bearing, activity helps keep bones stronger. *Move more today.*
- *Eat smarter.* Enjoy more fruits, vegetables, and whole-grain products, fewer high-fat foods, enough calcium-rich foods, and enough calories for a healthy weight. *Take one step toward smarter eating today.*

March 13   Move for a Worthy Cause

Get more from your workout than a workout! If you plan to walk, bike, run, swim, or some other active sport, why not do so for a worthy cause?

With spring around the corner, you'll see promotions for bike-a-thons, walk-a-thons, and dance-a-thons; many are fund-raisers to support worthy causes. Join in! Do it with friends or with family.

- *If you stay physically active,* look for an event that challenges you.
- *If you've been sitting through the winter,* find a fun event that's not too strenuous. Start moving now.
- *If you're a community volunteer,* organize some kind of "move-a-thon," even if it's just for a small group of local citizens or organization members.

March 14   Cook Savvy—Vitamins Are In

Your kitchen is stocked with vitamin-rich fruits and vegetables. Now, how do you get those nutrients to your dinner table? Store and prepare fruits and vegetables with care. Improper food storage and prep can leave some nutrients behind.

To keep more vitamins in, improve one or more of your culinary skills today.

- *Go under cover.* Cook fruits and veggies in a covered pot so nutrients that dissolve in water (B vitamins and vitamin C) don't disappear in steam.
- *Keep the "a-peel."* The edible peel, outer leaves, and area just below the peel contain many vitamins and minerals.
- *Skimp on water.* Better yet, steam, microwave, or stir-fry fruits and veggies, so water-soluble vitamins don't come in contact with water.
- *Cook fast*—just until tender-crisp. The shorter the cooking time, the less nutrients are loss. Besides, your veggies will look and taste better.
- *Enjoy raw flavor.* Heat destroys some B vitamins and vitamin C. So enjoy fruit and vegetables raw.

March 15   Weighty Problems

If you read health headlines, you know that obesity is today's top health epidemic. Why the alarm? Among other reasons, obesity has been cited as a major cause of death and disease, increasing the risks for heart disease, stroke, high blood pressure, diabetes, and some cancers. The risks are higher if excess body fat is around the abdomen.

Your charge: keeping your weight within a healthy range.

These five strategies all promote a healthy weight. Pick one. Then take action with small steps, starting today.

1. *Move more.* Build up to 60 minutes of moderate activity daily. Spend less leisure time sitting—watching TV, at the computer. You'll find lots of ways in this book.
2. *Eat more slowly.* Pay attention to know if you're really hungry and when you're full. See February 18.
3. *Try smaller portions.* Start with less. If you're really hungry, you can go back for more. See January 31.
4. *Enjoy five to nine fruit and vegetable servings a day.* Most are low in calories.
5. *Drink more water.* Consume fewer soft drinks.

March 16   "A" to Avocados

Though they aren't sweet, avocados are actually fruit, and they have unheralded health benefits. Avocados provide heart-healthy *folate; vitamins E, C,* and *B₆; potassium;* and *soluble fiber.* Their fat is mostly monounsaturated, the kind that's heart-healthy. And avocados have phytonutrient benefits: cholesterol-lowering *plant sterols; glutathione,* which works as an antioxidant potentially for cancer protection; and *lutein,* which promotes healthy vision.

Ripe avocados are slightly soft to pressure from your palm. Use them mashed as a spread, slivered and layered in sandwiches, or in a new recipe, such as this one:

Prosciutto-Salmon Wraps

2 avocados, seeded and peeled*	8 slices smoked salmon
8 slices prosciutto	Fresh lemon or lime, sliced

Cut each avocado into 8 slices. Diagonally wrap each with a prosciutto or salmon slice. Arrange wraps on serving platter, garnish with lemon or lime, and serve. Makes 4 (4-wrap) servings.

Source: California Avocado Commission
*Cut each avocado lengthwise around the seed. Rotate the halves to separate. Slide a spoon's tip gently under the seed; lift it out. To peel, place the cut side down, and remove skin with your fingers.

March 17   🍎 Go for Green

Wearing green for St. Patrick's Day? Why not make a meal to match? From broccoli and green beans to spinach and green peppers, count all the ways you can fill your plate with greens!

Properly prepared, green veggies add color appeal to your meals. Cooked just until tender-crisp, they add flavor appeal. Besides that, dark-green veggies supply plenty of nutrients—*vitamin C, folate,* and *vitamin K,* to name a few. Today we know they also supply two key *carotenoids*—lutein and zeaxanthin—which may promote eye health. And plant substances in greens may lower your risk for heart disease and some cancers, too.

Go green!

- *Think beyond the iceberg!* Vary your salad greens: use spinach, romaine, watercress, chicory, escarole.
- *Serve on a bed of greens.* Arrange grilled or roasted fish, chicken, or meat atop tender-crisp green beans or wilted spinach.
- *Get leafy.* Tuck chopped fresh spinach and other greens into sandwiches, pita, and wraps—and in lasagna, risotto, pasta dishes, and burritos.
- *Nosh on green snacks:* raw broccoli spears, asparagus spears, zucchini slices, or crisp snow peas.

March 18   🚶 Walk a Fit Line

Does physical activity take priority in your life? Or do busy schedules interfere? Consider this: Nearly everyone can fit walking into a lifestyle. And it pays off!

Warm up, then stretch first. Walk briskly; the faster you walk, the greater the benefits. Pump your arms. Wear good walking shoes. Bring your water bottle. Enjoy!

Now, walk your way to fitness!

- *Set a measurable goal.* If it's realistic, you won't give up.
- *Track your progress.* Drive to measure the distance, or get a pedometer to track every step. For fitness, try for at least 10,000 steps (about 3 miles) a day. (See January 30.)
- *Walk with a friend or your dog.* A walking buddy and a regular routine encourage stick-to-itiveness.
- *Pick a safe, interesting route.* Walk in a neighborhood with side-walks, a shopping mall, or a nearby park.
- *Schedule walking into your lifestyle.* Do it first thing before you get busy, during your lunch break, or after hours to clear your mind.
- *Reward your success.* Pick something that feeds your walking habit (fitness magazine, new walking shoes, a heart rate monitor, an audiotape to enjoy as you walk).

March 19   Safe for the Taking

If you "take out to eat in," your doggie bag or take-out meal poses a potential food safety risk. As the weather heats up, the risk soars higher.

To avoid the guessing game of doggie bag safety, follow this advice:

- *Chill promptly.* For take-out food and restaurant leftovers, that means within two hours. If the outdoor temperature swells to 90°F or more, store food within an hour.
- *Date it.* Label your doggie bag or take-out package. Eat what's inside within three to four days. Remember, spoiled food may not look, smell, or taste bad.
- *Reheat thoroughly.* Use a meat thermometer to check. The safe reheating temperature for restaurant or any leftovers is 165°F.

March 20   Using Your Noodles

Are you a noodle lover? Then celebrate National Noodle Month! Pasta, a mainly wheat product, is well known for its energy-producing complex carbs. Enriched and fortified, its *folic acid* helps prevent birth defects and may promote heart health, its *iron* protects against anemia, and its *B vitamins* help your body produce energy.

Those with celiac disease (gluten intolerance) or wheat allergies can find noodles that are made from other grains (barley, rice), beans, and starchy vegetables. Check the ingredient list to be sure wheat flour isn't used, too.

Consider so many pasta-bilities! Some hints to start: 1 pound of uncooked pasta equals 8 cups cooked pasta; tomato-based sauces usually have fewer calories and less fat than creamy white sauces.

- *Create your signature pasta dish* with this recipe "formula": 1 pound uncooked pasta + 4 cups vegetables + 2 to 3 cups cheese and/or lean meat, poultry, or fish + 1 to 2 cups sauce + $\frac{1}{4}$ to $\frac{1}{2}$ cup flavoring ingredients (fresh herbs, onion, other) + salt and pepper to taste. (Source: Adapted from National Pasta Association)
- *Make pasta primavera* with veggies of your choice to celebrate the upcoming start of spring. Use the recipe formula above. Slice and stir-fry fresh vegetables like these for your great pasta dish: asparagus, broccoli, carrots, bell pepper (red, orange, or green), green beans, mushrooms, spinach, tomato, zucchini, leftover veggies—whatever else you like!

March 21   Colorectal Cancer—Are You at Risk?

From age 50 on, everyone is at risk for colorectal cancer. Your risk is higher if you have a personal or family history of noncancerous colorectal polyps; colorectal cancer; inflammatory bowel disease; or ovarian, endometrial, or breast cancer.

The good news is that colorectal cancer is preventable.

National Colorectal Cancer Awareness Month is a good time to start reducing your risk.

- *Get tested.* If you're age 50 or at high risk, make an appointment for a colonoscopy. Detected early, polyps can be removed before they become cancerous.
- *Get physically active, or stay active.* Exercise may help reduce your risk.

- *Eat a low-fat diet, high in vegetables and fruits.* Although eating fruits and vegetables may not prevent colorectal cancer, their nutrients, fiber, and phytonutrients may help reduce the chances.
- *Enjoy more milk and other calcium-rich foods.* Consuming enough calcium is linked to colon cancer protection.

Three more strategies may offer protection: (1) take a multivitamin with folic acid, calcium, and vitamin D; (2) don't smoke; and (3) drink alcohol only in moderation, if at all.

March 22 In a Food Rut?

Are the same foods in heavy rotation at your house? Fact is, most people stick to their personal basics, planning meals around their same 10 to 15 core foods.

Eating a variety of foods is healthier, however. Why? Because each helps keep you healthy in a different way.

Defined in food terms, variety means eating many different foods (especially fruits, vegetables, and grain products) for their different nutrients, phytonutrients (plant substances), and other food substances. Consider: Plant-based foods have thousands of different phytonutrients; every fruit, vegetable, and grain product has a different line-up. For meat, poultry, fish, eggs, and dairy foods, there are plenty of nutritional differences, too!

Try one new food today when you:

- *Order from a restaurant menu.* Eating out is a perfect chance to experiment.
- *Shop in your local supermarket.* Check what's new to you in the produce department, the meat and seafood counter, the freezer case, the dairy department—even the canned food aisle. Buy one new food.
- *Leaf through a cookbook.* Cook an old favorite in a new way.

March 23 Just Add Five Plus Five

Want to make the most of a workout? Start with a 5- or 10-minute warm-up. Cool down with 5 more.

Warming up gradually gets your body systems geared up for high-intensity action. As your heart and breathing rates increase, more blood (and oxygen) flows to your muscles. Your core body temperature rises, warming your muscles. Your muscles and tendons become more flexible, with more range of motion.

Among the benefits? Your muscles contract faster and more forcefully, and you can work your muscles longer without discomfort. The chance for injury goes down.

Cooling down is important, too, to slowly reduce your heart rate and rid your muscles of lactic acid, which causes muscle fatigue. Properly done, you won't feel as tired after a workout. Stretching out muscle tightness helps reduce soreness later. Worth it!

When you get moving today, add 5 plus 5 minutes.

- *Start slowly with a 5-minute warm-up.* After your muscles are warmed up, gently stretch your large muscle groups: shoulders, arms, chest, elbows, calves, hamstrings, quadriceps, and knees. (See November 7.)
- *Work up to a brisk pace.*
- *Slow down with a 5-minute cool-down,* using your warm-up movements.

March 24 Eating in the Free-Way?

"Sugar-free," "fat-free," "cholesterol-free," "sodium-free," "trans-fat-free": How do you know if "freebie" foods are really a health bargain?

- *The label's Nutrition Facts and ingredient list tell more.* A fat-free food may have more sweetener than its traditional counterpart. Net result: The calories per serving may be equal.
- *Calories, even in fat-free foods, add up.* Portions bigger than label servings have more calories, too.
- *Any food needs to fit into the big picture.* Choose a calorie-free food to complement other food choices, not as an excuse to over-do on other foods.

If a "-free" food catches your eye today:

- *Turn to the Nutrition Facts.* To make it "-free" of something, one ingredient may be substituted for another; for example, a sugar-free food may be higher in fat, or vice versa. Buy smart!
- *Control your portion,* even if the food is fat-, calorie-, or cholesterol-free.

March 25 Passport to Health—Eating Greek Style

Celebrate Greek culinary traditions today on Greece's Independence Day!

If you stop at a Greek restaurant, try souvlaki (grilled lamb marinated in lemon juice, oil, and herbs), dolmas (stuffed vegetables), or a gyro (roasted, minced lamb with onion, bell peppers, and tzatziki sauce, stuffed in a pita). Go easy on vegetable pies (spanakopita), baba ghanouj (eggplant and olive oil), baklava (sweet walnut phyllo dessert), and olive oil dipping sauce. Their calories add up!

Prepare a simple Greek-inspired dish.

- *Create a Greek pizza.* Brush a pita with olive oil and top with feta cheese, plum tomatoes, olives, and herbs (oregano, rosemary, thyme)—then bake.
- *Toss a Greek salad.* Greens, garnished with black olives, feta cubes (just a few), tomato, and cucumber, are tossed with olive oil, lemon juice, and oregano. (For dressing, figure 2 parts olive oil, 1 part lemon juice.)
- *Enjoy a traditional Greek ending:* fresh fruit. Citrus is a favorite; try grapes or figs, too.

Tzatziki Salad with Tomato (in Garlic-Yogurt Dressing)

1 cup plain low-fat yogurt	2 cloves garlic, crushed
½ cup fresh mint, chopped fine	black pepper, to taste
½ cup fresh parsley, chopped fine	1 pound cucumbers (about 2
4 green onions, minced	medium), peeled and chopped
3 tablespoons lemon juice	½ pound tomatoes, chopped

Mix yogurt, mint, parsley, green onions, lemon juice, garlic, and pepper together. Pour over cucumber and tomato mixture, and toss. Serve within an hour for best taste. Makes 6 servings.

Source: Produce for Better Health Foundation

March 26   Your Weigh to Health

Is your inner voice telling you to trim or to gain a few pounds? What's a healthy, realistic weight—for *you?* "Right weight" is an individual matter that depends in part on your height, the size and shape of your body frame, and your muscle mass.

From a fitness standpoint, healthy weight is linked to your numbers: blood cholesterol, triglycerides, blood pressure, and fasting blood sugar levels. You can be fit at any size, *if* your numbers fall within a healthy range.

From a psychological standpoint, your healthy weight goal should be attainable and sensibly achieved. Even a few trimmed pounds can make a difference. An unrealistic approach that breeds failure isn't healthy for your psyche.

Get a handle on your best weight.

- *Find out your Body Mass Index (BMI)*—one indicator of a healthy weight. Go to www.cdc.gov/nccdphp/dnpa/bmi for a handy online calculator to figure it. If your BMI hits 25 or more, that might signal overweight.
- *Schedule a physical checkup* to learn if your numbers fall within a healthy range, whatever your weight or BMI.
- *Set a sensible weight goal* that's healthy and attainable for you.

March 27   Another Reason—Enjoy Fruit, Veggies, Grains

Do the benefits of enjoying plant-based foods seem endless? Their contribution of folate, a B vitamin essential for making new, healthy body cells, is one more reason, no matter what your age.

- *For anyone:* as protection from one form of anemia, which affects energy levels. Folate helps build red blood cells that carry oxygen to your cells to produce energy.
- *For women ages 14 to 50 (pregnant or not):* to reduce the risk for birth defects. If you have a chance of getting pregnant, it's essential insurance.

- *Again for anyone:* as a potential heart health benefit. A high level of homocysteine, an amino acid in blood, may suggest heart disease. Folate, and perhaps some other B vitamins, in food choices may help bring it down.

Enjoy grain products, fortified by law with folic acid (a form of folate). Add one more folate-rich fruit or vegetable serving to a meal today.

- *Enjoy spinach salad.* Toss in strawberries, or orange or grapefruit slices for more folate still.
- *Drink orange juice for breakfast.* OJ is rich in folate.
- *Snack on hummus,* made with folate-rich chickpeas. Go easy, because hummus has fat, too.
- *Eat breakfast cereal* fortified with folic acid. Read the label for how much.

March 28   Eggs-cellent!

Eggs are misperceived by many as a "forbidden" food. Today's research shows that one egg yolk a day is okay for most healthy people, as long as their total cholesterol intake comes in at 300 milligrams a day or less. (One large yolk has about 215 milligrams of cholesterol; egg whites are cholesterol free.)

Benefits: One large egg has just 70 calories. Yet it's a good source of *protein,* and a source of *vitamins A and D, B complex vitamins,* and *phosphorus.* Beyond that, eggs supply *lutein* and *zeaxanthin,* which may promote healthy vision.

Plan a meal around eggs. Here's an easy, nutrient-rich recipe to try!

Eggs Florentine Olé!

Cooking spray
1 10-ounce package frozen chopped spinach, thawed and well drained
4 eggs
¼ cup chunky salsa

¼ cup shredded reduced-fat Monterey Jack cheese
Sour half-and-half, reduced-fat sour cream, or additional salsa, if desired

Preheat oven to 325°F. Evenly coat four 6-ounce custard cups with cooking spray. Press spinach into coated cups. With back of spoon, make an indentation in center of spinach. Break and slip an egg into each indentation. Top each with 1 tablespoon salsa and 1 tablespoon cheese. Bake in oven until whites are completely set and yolks begin to thicken but are not hard, about 20 minutes. Top with sour half-and-half, if desired. Makes 4 servings.

Source: American Egg Board

March 29   Well-Come to Your Senses

How would you describe a perfect meal? By its sweet or savory flavor, its eye-appealing appearance, its mouth-watering aroma, its tender-crisp or silky-smooth texture, its important health benefits—or all five? A great meal creates a synergy of science *and* sensory appeal on your plate.

Try to blend flavor and health at your table.

- *Cook for eye appeal.* Substances that give leafy greens their deep-green color are good for your eyes, too. Colorful pigments in fruits and veggies also may protect you from heart disease, cancer, and other diseases.
- *Salt, but with a light touch.* From the entrée to dessert, salt enhances flavor in many healthful foods. Just go easy since it's high in sodium.
- *Cook with garlic.* Its pungent flavor and aroma come from phytonutrients that may protect against cancer and heart disease.
- *Flavor with citrus.* The ascorbic acid not only provides flavor balance; it's also a powerful antioxidant.
- *Marinate with yogurt.* Yogurt's friendly bacteria not only tenderize poultry and impart tart flavor; they also may promote immunity, may reduce symptoms of lactose intolerance, and may help protect you from some cancers and high blood cholesterol.

March 30   Confronting the "Weekend Warrior"

Do you spring into action on warm-weather weekends with a vigorous workout in the garden or on a bike—then awaken Monday feeling exhausted and sore?

No question, a physically active weekend is good for you. But staying active throughout the week, throughout the seasons is far better. From weight management, strength training, and bone health to blood pressure control, heart health, and cancer protection, the many health benefits come only from a regular physical activity routine. With a regular routine come stamina and strength, so your weekend workouts don't leave you hurting.

Try this to confront "weekend warriorism":

- *Start moving more today.* Even just 15 minutes of brisk walking offers health benefits. Work up to 60!
- *Be realistic* if you've been inactive. Skip the urge to overdo.
- *Warm up your muscles, then stretch.* Especially when you've been inactive, your muscles are tight, and your injury risk is high.

March 31   Motiv-action

Did your New Year start with a zeal for fitness? Great! Have you stuck with it? When life gets busy or stressful, staying motivated gets tough.

Truth is, motivation comes from inside, with the mental drive to act on something that's important to you. No one can do that for you. Overcome the barriers—and stay motivated.

- *Rethink your goals.* Set new, realistic, achievable ones. You can enjoy a competitive run, but you don't need to win.
- *Form a partnership.* Whether it's eating smarter or moving more, staying motivated is easier with a companion. And a partner's enthusiasm can be contagious!
- *Post a motivational quote.* A reminder on your fridge, bulletin board, or mirror may help keep you focused. Perhaps "Take ten, whenever you can!" (10 minutes of physical activity six times daily).
- *Give yourself an incentive.* Sometimes sticking with it is its own reward. But if not, treat yourself to a day spa, a concert ticket, or whatever "pushes your go button"!

April 1   🍴 No Fooling!

"Vitamin E *cures* cancer." "A grapefruit diet *guarantees* weight loss." "Fish oil *prevents* arthritis." Believe it? April Fools!

Who doesn't want an easy way to fitness, weight loss, or health? The trouble is, long-term health goals can't be reached with short-term quackery. In fact, misleading advice can harm you, especially if it overrides sound advice from reliable health experts.

Be shrewd so you're not misled by baffling nutrition claims.

- *Skip guarantees and promises.* Few things in life are surefire. Move on.
- *Watch out for miracles and magic.* Terms such as "cure," "effortless," "secret," and "miraculous" are hype, not sound science.
- *Seek an expert.* If a claim goes against the guidance of most respected health organizations, chances are it's quackery. For sound nutrition advice, find a registered dietitian. (See March 1.)
- *Be sensible.* The key to healthful eating is simple: a variety of food, in moderation (not too much, especially fat, saturated fat, added sugars, and salt), chosen with balance. Read January 15 and 16 again for guidelines; find simple strategies throughout this book.

April 2   🍎 Soy Smart

When you grocery shop, do you see "soy" everywhere? With more known about its benefits, soy has become a popular ingredient in foods, from cereals to sausages!

A few benefits? For one, about 25 grams of soy protein a day may help lower your cholesterol. Even less may lower cancer risk. What's more, soybeans have phytoestrogens that may help protect you from hormone-related cancers (breast or prostate)—and if you're female, from hot flashes during menopause or bone loss afterward.

It's National Soy Foods Month! For "soy good" nutrition and flavor, reach for soy-rich foods (not just supplements).

- *Enjoy soy beverages* on cereal, in cooking, in smoothies. If you limit cow's milk, get a calcium- and vitamin B_{12}-fortified soy beverage.
- *Use soft and silken tofu* in place of ricotta cheese in lasagna, or in place of sour cream in dips.
- *Try firm tofu, tempeh, or soyburgers.* Their firm texture works great in casseroles, stir-fries, soups, and stews—or any meat or poultry dish.
- *Snack on soy.* Try edamame (fresh soybeans shelled or in the pod), a soy snack bar, soynuts (¼ cup soynuts has 200 calories and 10 fat grams; go easy).

April 3   Advice—Bound to Put You to Sleep

Want to accomplish more in your day? Handle everyday stress better? Improve your memory? Perhaps you need more sleep.

Lifestyle choices, stress, and sleep disorders have turned America into a culture of sleeplessness. Although most American adults sleep less than seven hours daily, research shows that eight hours offer more benefits. In addition, preliminary medical research suggests a lack of sleep may be linked to heart disease, hypertension, lowered immunity, obesity, and neurological disorders.

Sleep tight starting now—it's National Sleep Awareness Week.

To get the benefits from a full night's sleep:

- *Make your surroundings sleep friendly:* darkened quiet room, comfortable surface and pillow, cool temperature.
- *Move more during the day,* but not too close to bedtime. Exercise "pumps up" your metabolism for several hours.
- *Time any stimulants.* If you're caffeine sensitive, avoid caffeinated drinks for six to eight hours before bedtime. Skip smoking, too.
- *Skip a late-night drink.* Alcoholic drinks before bedtime interfere with and may interrupt deep, restful sleep.
- *Get into a sleep routine.* Go to sleep and wake up at the same time every day.

April 4 ✍ Spring Clean Your Fridge

Spring cleaning your household? Remember the refrigerator!

Appliances collect food debris that harbors harmful bacteria. If the inside fridge temperature exceeds 40°F—common as outdoor temperature rises—the likelihood of harmful bacteria increases.

Put your fridge on your cleaning schedule today.

- *Check your owner's manual.* For efficiency and the best cooling, find out how to clean the front grill and the condenser coils. Unplug the refrigerator when you clean the coils.
- *Scrub the whole inside*—shelves, drawers, freezer. Use a clean sponge and warm soapy water, rinse with clean water, then dry with a clean cloth or paper towel.
- *Wipe up spills immediately,* especially raw meat, poultry, and fish juices.
- *Sort weekly.* Toss any foods past their prime. Check expiration dates. When in doubt, throw out.
- *Eliminate odors.* Keep an open box of baking soda on a back shelf; change it every three months.
- *Buy a refrigerator thermometer for the center of the middle shelf.* Adjust fridge settings so the temp stays below 40°F.

April 5 🚶 Green Thumbs Up for Gardening

Digging, raking, bending, hauling. Want a satisfying way to be more active if sports don't appeal? A garden might be just your thing.

How Yard Work Stacks Up as an Energy Burner

| | If you weigh | |
| | 120 pounds | 170 pounds |
Activity	Calories burned per hour	
gardening	275	385
lawn mowing (not on a sit-down mower)	300	425
brisk walking around the neighborhood	220	310
housework	135	190
sitting in the garden	55	75

Make today a gardening day.

- *Start spring cleanup.* Rake, turn the soil, remove debris.
- *Dig a new garden bed.* Plant savory herbs, tender lettuce, or succulent vegetables.
- *Haul and spread*—compost, top soil, mulch.
- *Cut or fertilize your lawn.*

April 6 Supplements and Meds—A Dangerous Mix

Are you taking over-the-counter or prescription medicine? Dealing with a chronic health problem? Preparing for surgery? If so, be especially cautious of supplements.

Supplement-medication combos may interfere with or boost the effect of medication to harmful levels. Either way, their interaction may become dangerous.

Consider some examples:

- Vitamin E, garlic, ginkgo biloba, as well as aspirin and Coumadin (prescription drug) *all* thin blood.
- St. John's wort can make oral contraceptives, as well as prescription drugs for treating heart disease, depression, certain cancers, or seizures, less effective.
- Ephedra (in some weight-loss products), garlic, ginkgo, kava, St. John's wort, and valerian can change your heart rate and blood pressure and increase bleeding—risky for surgery.

If you choose to use supplements, protect your health.

- *Listen for health alerts.* The U.S. Food and Drug Administration issues advisories about products causing adverse reactions.
- *Let your doctor and pharmacist know!* Talk about any supplements you take, especially if you're having surgery, taking any medication, or dealing with a health problem. (Probably stop any supplement at least two to three weeks before elective surgery.)

April 7   Let-tuce Keep You Healthy

Next to potatoes, lettuce is the most popular veggie in the United States. Which leafy greens go into your salads?

Dark-green leafy greens offer plenty of the antioxidant *beta carotene* (forms vitamin A), which may help protect you from cancer and may slow aging, and another antioxidant, *vitamin C*. The darker the leaves, the more nutrient-rich the lettuce. (Romaine has seven times more vitamin A and C than iceberg lettuce.) Some greens deliver *folate, potassium,* and *fiber,* too. Greens supply *lutein,* which contributes to good vision and may help protect your eyes from cataracts and macular degeneration. And leafy greens fill a plate with few calories and essentially no fat (except what's added with dressing).

Perk up your salad making—more flavor, color, texture—by mixing in different greens.

- *For a peppery flavor:* arugula or watercress
- *For leaves that aren't green:* red-and-white radicchio
- *For flavor with a "bite":* chicory or escarole
- *For a mild flavor and delicate green color:* mache or Boston or Bibb lettuce
- *For a deep-green color:* spinach
- *For a crisp texture:* Romaine

April 8   Have a Spa Day

Need a chance to rejuvenate and de-stress your life? Rather than splurge at an expensive resort spa, luxuriate with a spa day at home. Invite your friends.

At-home spa tips:

- *Create the space:* a quiet spot, comfortable chairs and pillows, gentle music, aromatic candles.
- *Fill baskets with spa products:* moisturizers, facial creams, massage lotions, fragrances, nail polish, pumice stone, and more.

- *Invite guests:* Suggest they bring comfortable clothes and walking shoes. Take turns giving massages, manicures, and facials. Consider hiring a massage therapist.
- *Plan and prepare simple, flavorful "spa food" from your home kitchen.*
  - Fruit, vegetables, legumes, whole-grain foods—in mixed salads, pasta or rice dishes, light soups, fruit smoothies, more
  - Low-fat ingredients and cooking: perhaps grilled vegetables, herb-roasted chicken salad, seared salmon, broiled fish tacos, yogurt dips
  - Refreshing drinks: green tea, juice, fruit smoothies, sparkling water
  - Sensible portions—with a plate that's at least two-thirds veggies, fruit, and whole-grain foods and one-third animal-based foods. Try tapa-size portions.

April 9   Cook Savvy—More Calcium, Great Flavor

It's well known that calcium is a bone builder. Calcium-rich foods may also help protect you from colon cancer and high blood pressure, as well as osteoporosis, and they may play a role in weight control. Getting the recommended two to three servings of calcium-rich dairy foods is easy.

Try a quick-and-easy calcium booster.

- *Add a slice of flavor.* Try a unique cheese—grated Asiago on grilled vegetables or hearty soup, dilled havarti with salmon, or gorgonzola with crisp apple or pear slices.
- *Whirl a "more-than-fruit" smoothie.* Blend milk, yogurt, or a calcium-fortified soy beverage with your favorite fruits.
- *Fortify!* Blend in a little plain yogurt, grated cheese, or milk with mashed potatoes.

Pecan-Cherry Yogurt Dip

1 cup plain yogurt
3 tablespoons honey
¼ cup chopped pecans

¼ cup chopped dry cherries or
   cranberries

In a medium bowl, stir yogurt and honey together. Mix in pecans and cherries. Cover and refrigerate until serving. Makes 1½ cups dip.

April 10   Pass the Color-Crunch Test?

When you think nutrition, think taste. A healthful meal nourishes only if it's appealing enough for you to eat!

Some qualities that make meals so appealing also add health-promoting value. Fruits and vegetables with different colors offer different nutrients and phytonutrients: *orange* sweet potatoes, *deep-yellow* mango, *red* tomatoes, *dark-green* spinach, and *purple* grapes. Vegetables cooked just until they're tender-crisp retain more valuable vitamins. Hearty whole-grain breads, often chewier, contain more fiber.

Put variety and appeal on your menu today.

- *Add a colorful fruit or vegetable.* Looks great, and good for you!
- *Cook your vegetables just until tender-crisp* for more color, better texture, and more nutrition.
- *Spark it up with a garnish.* Even a citrus slice, an herb sprig, or a few toasted nuts make ordinary dishes look more appealing.

April 11   Take Me Out to the Ball Game

Whether during the first inning or the seventh-inning stretch, chances are you'll get hungry during a three-hour major-league ball game.

Traditional choices abound: hot dogs, beer, popcorn. The good news is that today's ballpark fare just might include some surprising options, from crab cakes or sushi to low-fat frozen yogurt or fresh fruit cups—and water.

If you head to the ballpark now that the baseball season's open:

- *Eat something first.* That takes the edge off your hunger so you won't overdo on high-fat, high-calorie ballpark foods.
- *Know your food options.* Decide before you line up to buy. As a regular fan, scope out the offerings early in the season. If you take in just a game or two a season, call a fan for the insider food story.
- *Go easy on beer and other alcoholic drinks.* Calories add up. Plus, you may need to drive home after the game.

- *Take your seventh-inning stretch.* Walk around the stadium, up and down the ramps.
- *Drink plenty of water and use your sunscreen* if you're sitting out in the sun all day.
- *Enjoy the game.* If you do splurge on ballpark food, cut back the next day.

April 12   🜚 Apple or Pear?

We're talking about your body shape, not your favorite fruit! Why does it matter? An apple-shaped body may be riskier for your health than a pear shape.

- *Apple shape:* Even if your Body Mass Index (BMI) falls within a healthy range, abdominal or upper body fat increases risks for diabetes, high cholesterol levels, early heart disease, and high blood pressure. (See January 23.)
- *Pear shape:* Extra weight below the waist—hips, buttocks, thighs—may be less risky for most health problems, except for varicose veins and orthopedic problems.

Your genes, gender, and age affect where your body stores fat. Men tend to store more around the middle; with a menopausal hormone shift, many women may store more fat there, too.

A tape measure will tell you what "shape" you're in.

- *Standing, measure just above your hipbone.* Relax, and breathe out when you measure. Don't cinch in the tape measure or pull in your stomach.
- *Judge your risk.* It goes up with waist size: higher if your waist measures more than 35 inches for a woman or more than 40 inches for a man.

April 13   ✍ Passport to Health—Eating Thai Style

In Thailand, the Songkran celebration brings in the New Year with ritual water-throwing fun—and flavorful food! Among Thai cuisine's signature ingredients are lemongrass, peanuts—and hot-hot chilies!

If you enjoy eating at a Thai restaurant today, try pad thai (stir-fried noodle dish), tom yum koong (broth-based soup), or spring rolls in rice paper. Go easy on fried menu options or curries made with coconut milk. Their calories can add up.

Another option: Prepare a Thai-inspired dish at home.

Thai-Style Beef Salad

1 pound lean beef sirloin steak (½ inch thick), fat-trimmed
2 tablespoons reduced-sodium soy sauce
2 tablespoons rice vinegar
1 tablespoon lemon juice
1½ teaspoons brown sugar
1 clove garlic, minced

1 teaspoon sesame oil
¼ teaspoon red pepper flakes
4 cups shredded lettuce
1½ cups shredded carrots
1 cup thinly sliced green onions
1 cup cooked thin spaghetti (2 ounces dry)
¼ cup cilantro leaves, loosely packed

Cut beef into strips 2 inches long by ¼ inch thick. In a large nonstick skillet, stir-fry beef strips over high heat until brown, about 3 minutes. Remove from pan; cool to room temperature. To make dressing, in a small bowl mix soy sauce, vinegar, lemon juice, brown sugar, garlic, sesame oil, and red pepper flakes; set aside. In a large bowl combine beef with lettuce, carrots, green onions, cooked spaghetti, and cilantro; toss with reserved dressing. Serve immediately. Makes 4 servings.

Source: Produce for Better Health Foundation

April 14   Move on the Cheap

Do high costs cramp your fitness style? You don't have to spend hundreds on gym memberships or equipment to stay fit. All you may need is a good pair of walking shoes.

To move on the cheap:

- *Turn household objects into workout weights.* Start by weight-lifting 15-ounce cans of food. Work up to gallon milk jugs (8 pounds).
- *Walk rather than drive if your destination is close.* You'll save on gas money, too. Get a small daypack to carry things easily.
- *Pump up the tires in your (or your kid's) bike. Get rolling* instead of buying a stationary cycle or fancy mountain bike.

- *Dig, plant, and care for a vegetable garden.* You'll exercise and save on and savor a little home-grown produce.

April 15   Tax Day—Stressless Eating

Racing to finish your taxes? Stressed by the tax-dollar bottom line? Besides zapping energy and perhaps making you irritable, stress can contribute to health costs: headaches, hypertension, lower immunity, muscle tension, sleeplessness.

How do you manage stress so it doesn't manage you? Abusing food—either obsessive eating or meal skipping—to deal with stress makes no sense. A moderate approach, with a variety of foods, works better. You get needed nourishment to deal with this frenzied world, and you up your chances to stay healthy and keep your weight normal.

Make time today to downsize personal stress.

- *Set goals; prioritize.* Jot down what's really important to you (skip "shoulds"). Prioritize your goals: top, middle, low. Can "low" ones go?
- *Give yourself some space.* Take a 10-minute break, then reassess.
- *Let go.* Find at least one thing today that you don't need to do; repeat that tomorrow, and the next day. Get the idea?
- *Binge no more.* If you're tempted to eat when you're stressed, list five other things you could do instead: take a bubble bath, read a good book, garden. Do one as your stress antidote!
- *Put your body in gear.* Physical activity is often a great stress reliever.

April 16   Catch the Volunteer Spirit

Do you take time to volunteer? As a lifelong habit, volunteering your time and effort may be worth even more than you think.

In one study, just 40 hours of volunteer time yearly for retired people tended to prolong life. In another, volunteers tended to be happier, more energetic, and in better control of their lives than nonvolunteers. Giving of yourself—no matter what your age—pays off in the positive mental energy that goes with giving.

As National Volunteer Week approaches, consider volunteering in a service, perhaps one that relates to food.

- *A community soup kitchen or food pantry,* which provides food for the needy
- *Your child's or grandchild's school cafeteria or after-school program,* where adult volunteers can help encourage healthful eating
- *A senior center,* where you take time to enjoy a meal with an older adult
- *A cause walk,* where you walk to raise funds for a cause, perhaps for a food pantry or the cause of your choice

April 17   24-Carrot Health

Did you know that feathery fresh carrot tops were worn to adorn hair in Shakespeare's day?

Today it's carrots' vibrant orange pigment, known as *carotene,* that's getting attention. Beta carotene turns into vitamin A, a powerful antioxidant vitamin. New research suggests that carrots' carotenoids may also reduce cancer risk, slow aging, and reduce some diabetes-related symptoms. In farmer's markets, heirloom carrots—scarlet, maroon, golden yellow, purple—are showing up, contributing still other antioxidants (such as anthocyanins in purple carrots).

Enjoy carrots today—as an easy finger food or prepared as an easy side dish.

Heart-Healthy Glazed Gingered Carrots

1 pound carrots, peeled and cut into ¼-inch slices
1 tablespoon margarine
2 tablespoons brown sugar
1 teaspoon ground ginger (or ½ teaspoon grated fresh ginger)
2 tablespoons fresh, finely chopped parsley

Steam carrots for 10 to 15 minutes, or until barely tender. In a medium-size frying pan, melt margarine until it bubbles. Add carrots and toss. Sprinkle with sugar and ginger. Toss lightly to coat carrots and continue cooking until carrots are lightly glazed, about 1 to 2 minutes. Just before serving, sprinkle with parsley. Makes 5 servings.

Source: Produce for Better Health Foundation

April 18   Let's Do Lunch

What are you doing for lunch today? Why not use your lunch break to do something that moves you, too? An active midday work break is not only good for your body; it's good for your head and may even boost your productivity.

Fit more active time into your workday.

- *Walk to lunch.* Pick an eating spot that's a 10- to 15-minute walk from work.
- *Keep walking shoes handy in your car or desk.* Now, no excuses to sit out your lunch break!
- *Hold walking meetings*—if you need to work through lunch.
- *Join a fitness center near work.* Schedule time on your business calendar to work out before or after work, or during your lunch break.
- *Remember to have lunch—even if you must eat deskside occasionally!*

April 19   Juicy Ideas

Do fruit drinks have the same nourishment you expect from fruit juice?

Only "100 percent juice" means full fruit nutrition. "Juice drinks" and "juice cocktails" are diluted juice, perhaps fortified, with added sweeteners that may boost calories. That said, tart juices, such as cranberry, need a little sweetener or diluting to taste good. And "fruit drinks" are basically flavored waters that lack full fruit nutrition, even if they're nutrient fortified.

Fruit juice—your best choice—contains its naturally present nutrients and phytonutrients. That can be a hefty amount of vitamins C and A daily. Juice with pulp has a little more fiber, but not as much as fruit itself. Fortified juice is okay, but calcium-fortified juice can't replace all of milk's nutrients.

For smart juice drinking:

- *Check the label.* The ingredient list shows if it's 100% juice, if it contains juice plus other ingredients, or if it's mostly water and sweetener. Nutrition Facts give nutrition specifics in a serving.
- *Enjoy, but don't overdo.* Go easy on juice or juice drinks. Up to 12 ounces daily is probably enough, because their calories add up.
- *Watch out!* Fruit-flavored drinks can't substitute for real juice.

April 20   "Veg Out"

You've heard: Eat "five to nine a day" veggies and fruits—three to five vegetable and two to four fruit servings daily. Why? Vegetables and fruits are:

- *Low in calories and fat* (unless fried or drizzled with butter, creamy sauce, or high-fat dressing). Their fats are mostly unsaturated, so healthier for your heart.
- *Cholesterol free,* like all plant sources of food
- *Good sources of many health-promoting vitamins and minerals,* perhaps beta carotene (vitamin A), folate, vitamin C, and potassium
- *Loaded with antioxidants, fiber, and other phytonutrients,* many with heart-healthy and cancer-protective benefits

Vegetarian or not, try a quick veggie "sandwich" for a great-tasting lunch!

- *Stack a TLT sandwich:* tofu, lettuce, and tomato on whole-wheat bread, flavored with onion, horseradish, and a splash of balsamic vinegar.
- *Bake a mushroom pita pizza:* sliced mushrooms, tomato, artichoke hearts, and pine nuts, drizzled with lemon juice and olive oil on a pita, topped with mozzarella.
- *Enjoy a grilled veggie "sub" or panini.* Tip: Portabella mushrooms give a meaty flavor.

April 21   "Soul" Food

What foods bring you comfort? Meatloaf and mashed potatoes? Pizza with the "works"? Mom's lasagna? Likely some foods enjoyed during your youth conjure up warm, soothing feelings. There's no specific list of comfort foods. We each have our own.

So, is indulging in comfort foods okay? Sure – *if* it doesn't lead to emotional overeating, *if* you also deal with negative emotions positively and away from food, and *if* it isn't all the time. If these foods are high fat, high calorie, or low in nutrients, certainly go easy.

When you reach for comfort foods, enjoy them in moderation.

- *Boost their value.* Add vegetables, fruits, whole grains, and beans—easier if pizza, chili, spaghetti, or many other mixed entrées are your comfort foods.
- *Savor the comfort from small portions,* especially if the food is high in calories or fat.
- *Update comfort foods for nutrition and convenience.* Perhaps substitute ground turkey in meatloaf, reduced-fat cheese in lasagna, refrigerated whole-wheat pizza crust topped with lots of veggies.

April 22   Second Time Around

Your resources count! This Earth Day celebrate your health and the planet's health by properly storing and creatively using leftovers.

Refrigerate leftovers: within two hours if they're at room temperature; one hour if the temperature is 90°F or more. Put leftovers in shallow pans so they chill faster.

Use refrigerated leftovers within a safe time.

- *Cooked vegetables, meat, poultry, and fish:* 3 to 4 days
- *Cooked seafood:* 2 days
- *Cooked pasta:* 3 to 5 days
- *Cooked rice:* 1 week
- *Cooked stuffing, gravy, and meat broth:* 1 to 2 days

Safely reheat meat, poultry, and fish leftovers to 165°F. Use a meat thermometer to check.

Turn yesterday's leftovers into a new dish.

- *Make convenience soup heartier.* Chop leftovers; toss them in as you heat the soup.
- *Cook a quiche or a frittata.* Mix leftovers in the egg mixture. Check a recipe for cooking directions.

April 23 🍎 Nuts about Almonds

In a nutshell, just a single ounce of almonds (20 to 25 almonds) is flavor-packed, convenient, and good for you. (See March 8.) Here's what's inside:

- *Vitamin E:* protection from cancer, heart disease, and cataracts. (*Tip:* You get one-third of a day's vitamin E from an ounce of almonds.)
- *Folate:* heart-health benefits, too, and it helps prevent birth defects.
- *Calcium, phosphorus, and magnesium:* a bone-building trio. Calcium and magnesium offer protection from hypertension, too.
- *Fiber:* an aid for digestion, it protects against cancer, heart disease, and other health problems, too.
- *Monosaturated fats:* the type of fat linked to less heart disease risk. *Bonus:* Almonds are cholesterol-free!

Three simple ways to enjoy almonds:

- *For a smoothie idea,* blend in one tablespoon of toasted almonds for every cup of smoothie.
- *For a crunchy almond butter,* process whole almonds with a touch of vegetable oil, salt, and sugar until nearly smooth.
- *For an easy add-in,* toss slivered almonds on stir-fries, salads, and rice, or sprinkle on cereal, veggies, fish, yogurt, or ice cream.

Spicy Cajun Almonds

2 teaspoons dried basil	½ teaspoon salt
1½ teaspoons garlic powder	½ teaspoon finely ground black
1 teaspoon dried thyme	pepper
1 teaspoon dried cayenne pepper	1 egg white
1 teaspoon paprika	2 cups whole almonds

Preheat oven to 325°F. Blend seasonings well. In a large bowl whisk egg white until opaque and frothy. Add almonds; toss to coat. Add seasonings; toss gently to coat evenly. Oil a baking sheet or coat with vegetable cooking spray. Arrange almonds on baking sheet in single layer. Bake for 15 minutes. Gently toss almonds; rearrange in single layer. Bake for another 15 minutes; toss gently. Turn off oven. Leave almonds in oven with door ajar for 15 minutes. Remove from oven; cool. Store in airtight container up to two weeks. Makes about 2 cups.

Source: Courtesy of the Almond Board of California, www.AlmondsAreIn.com

April 24 Indulge Success, Not Failure

Ever hear your inner voice say, "I always gain weight back, so what's the use of dieting?"

Thinking you'll fail—even before you try—breeds nearly surefire failure. Instead, put a positive mental spin on the past. If you tried and failed, and perhaps tried and failed again, you've already taken the first step toward change. That step? Awareness!

Now, take your next steps—overcome the barriers.

- *Reverse your thinking.* Visualize success, not failure, as a mental first step.
- *Learn from past failures.* What didn't work for you? What could you do differently? Jot down your ideas for healthier eating or living.
- *Remember your successes, too.* Indulge in positive thinking, even small victories. Nothing breeds success more than success.

April 25 Allergies—or Not?

With pollen in the spring air, thoughts often turn to allergies. Now's as good a time as any to address food allergies, too.

Though only about 2 to 2.5 percent of American adults have any type of food allergy, many more think they do. One reason for the discrepancy: self-diagnosis.

Most symptoms of food allergies are just uncomfortable. But in rare cases they can be severe, even life-threatening. So a medical diagnosis is wise, if for no other reason than peace of mind.

If you think you have a food allergy, get a medical opinion. Make an appointment and prepare for the visit.

- *Keep track.* Record your symptoms and what you ate or drank before they occurred.
- *Get your family history.* Did or does anyone else have allergies, including food allergies?
- *Record the bigger picture.* Does anything else, perhaps physical activity or drinking alcoholic beverages, bring symptoms on?

April 26   Beyond French Fries

Americans may be eating more vegetables today, but a significant percent of those veggies are French fries—more than 25 pounds per person yearly!

Potatoes do offer plenty of health benefits: *vitamin C, potassium,* and *fiber.* Fry that same potato and calories double, vitamin C drops by half, and fat gets added.

- *Challenge one:* A serving of fries (about 10) with 160 calories and 8 fat grams can fit with smart eating. However, most folks eat bigger portions.
- *Challenge two:* Potatoes aren't the only vegetable. They won't deliver all the health-promoting plant substances in green, deep-yellow, orange, and red fruits and vegetables. Variety is key.

Follow the five- to nine-a-day guideline with a simple edit: Eat at least five *different* fruit and vegetable servings today.

- *Pair fast food with salad.* Skip fries; order a garden salad, slaw, or fruit cup with your burger.
- *Pack whole fruit in your lunch bag.* Try a tangerine, kiwi, berries, not just an apple or banana. Or tuck in a can of single-serve fruit.
- *Add a veggie.* Enjoy one more vegetable (in a starter, salad, soup, side dish) than usual at dinner if you don't already consume at least three vegetable servings daily.

April 27   Child's Play

Have you played tag lately? Shot a few hoops? Jumped rope? Child's play makes great physical activity for grown-ups, too. Even more important, it's great family time and your chance to show that active living is healthful living at every age.

Actually, child's play teaches plenty! As kids climb, twist, jump, and run, their bodies get stronger, more coordinated, more flexible. They learn how to cooperate and share with playmates. Active play also can teach, develop the body-mind connection, and build self-confidence.

Other benefits? Active kids may sleep better, learn a positive way to release stress, and reduce their chance for overweight and type 2 diabetes. (*Tip:* Play along, and you'll get the same benefits; besides, it's a fun way to wind down your day.)

Fit child's play into your family's day.

- *Enjoy a playground together.* Equipment should be sturdy enough so you can swing, teeter-totter, or slide, too.
- *Play a pick-up game:* basketball, softball, sidewalk tennis.
- *Set aside play space* where it's okay and safe to tumble, jump, run, and kick a ball.

April 28   Savvy Kitchen—Nine Great Health-Wise Utensils

Shopping for a wedding or Mother's Day gift? Kitchen tools that help prepare healthful meals quickly and easily might be the perfect solution.

Shop for a "health-smart" cooking utensil today.

- *Blender or food processor* for blending fruit and yogurt smoothies
- *Coffee grinder* for grinding nuts, seeds, grains, dry herbs, and spices
- *Fat-separating pitcher* for pouring off broth and leaving fat behind

- *Instant-read thermometer* to quickly check for safe internal temperatures of cooked meat, poultry, fish, and leftovers
- *Indoor grill* to let fat drip away when cooking meat or poultry (good for grilling veggies, too)
- *Nonstick pots and pans* for cooking with little or no added fat
- *Pump spray bottle* to lightly spray poultry, fish, or baked goods with any oil you like
- *Ribbed frying pan* to let meat and poultry cook above fat drippings
- *Steamer* for no-fat cooking of vegetables, fish, or chicken

April 29   Stoke Your Appetite

Underweight? If so, you're probably tired of hearing people say how lucky you are.

Being too thin can be risky to your health. You need the fat layer just under your skin to help protect you from cold and cushion your body from injury. That fat layer is a source of stored energy if you need it. If underweight comes from undereating, the chances of tiredness, irritability, lack of concentration, and the risk of infection go up.

If you need to gain weight, do it smart. Eat plenty of nutrient-rich foods (but still without too much fat). Try frequent meals and snacks; drink beverages 30 minutes before and after eating, not with meals (so they don't fill you up); and yes, fit in physical activity, which builds muscle and stimulates appetite.

If you have a poor appetite for any reason including illness, fatigue, stress, medication, or disease—even if you're normal weight—try this to stimulate your appetite and make eating more appealing:

- *Eat five or six smaller meals* instead of three bigger ones during the day.
- *Add more appeal to food* with more color, more texture, more aroma in your meal.
- *Eat with friends.*

- *Drink a small glass of wine or beer before eating.*
- *Slow down.* If rushing takes your appetite away, plan stressful activities away from mealtime.
- *Walk before mealtime.*

April 30   Give Us the Berries

Bright red color, sweet, succulent flavor—do field-fresh strawberries conjure up wonderful sense-ations of spring?

Strawberries are among nature's best source of *vitamin C*, a vitamin that promotes immunity, lessens cold symptoms, and helps your body use iron. This antioxidant vitamin may offer heart-healthy and cancer-protective benefits, too. Strawberries also deliver *potassium, magnesium,* and some *folate.*

There's more: Strawberries contain plant substances (phytonutrients), including *quercetin, ellagic acid, anthocyanins,* and *kaempferol,* that may help protect you from cancer and heart disease, among others. All that for just 36 calories in 10 strawberries!

Enjoy strawberries in a new way today.

Fresh Strawberry Relish

2 tablespoons balsamic vinegar	½ teaspoon red pepper flakes
2 tablespoons orange juice	1 pint strawberries, stemmed and
1 tablespoon Dijon-style mustard	sliced
1 tablespoon honey	3 tablespoons raisins
½ teaspoon grated orange peel	3 tablespoons chopped walnuts

In medium bowl measure all ingredients except strawberries, raisins, and walnuts. Whisk to blend thoroughly. Add remaining ingredients; toss. Serve with baked or grilled fish or chicken. Makes 4 servings (about 1¾ cups).
Source: California Strawberry Commission

May 1   Bouquet on Your Plate

Ever tasted a pansy blossom, a rose petal, or a lily bud? Each adds a colorful garnish and distinctive flavor. Eat flowers? Perhaps you already enjoy capers (flower buds), saffron (blossom stigma), herb blossoms, and artichokes or broccoli (immature flowers).

This May Day, why not plant a bouquet of culinary flowers to enjoy this season? Try edible spring flowers such as pansies, violas, or violets in salads, crisp lilac fritters, or chicken salad spooned into a tulip.

Just be cautious! Avoid eating toxic species such as buttercup, daffodil, foxglove, lily of the valley, and sweet pea. If you're unsure, ask your county Extension agent (listed in your phone book's government pages). In any case, grow your own; flowers from the florist or greenhouse may have harmful chemicals.

Need fragrant ideas? Try:

- *Marigold and chrysanthemum petals* for color in salads, soups, seafood, or egg dishes
- *Nasturtiums* for peppery flavor in salads and pasta
- *Day lilies or squash blossoms* in stir-fries or sweet soup
- *Sweet rose or minty bee balm petals* in water or on puddings, ice cream, other sweet desserts
- *Lavender buds* to perfume lemonade, fruit salads, vinegar, cookies, sweet breads

May 2   Walk Your Talk, Talk Your Walk

You've heard this fitness advice: try to fit 60 minutes of *moderate* physical activity into your day. Fine, but what's moderate? Moderate activity isn't a leisurely stroll. From a numbers' standpoint, it adds up to the energy you burn by walking 2 miles in 30 minutes. That's about 150 calories, or about 1,000 calories weekly.

What else is considered "moderate"? Thirty minutes of fast dancing, water aerobics, leaf raking, or bicycling at 5 miles per hour all provide similar health and energy-burning benefits. So does washing and waxing a car for 45 to 60 minutes, washing windows or floors for 15 to 60 minutes, or gardening for 30 to 45 minutes.

To see if you get the benefits of moderate activity, take the "talk-sing" test when you're moving today:

- *Can you sing while you move?* Step up your pace!
- *Too breathless to talk?* Then slow down.
- *Can you talk as you move?* You're moving at a safe pace for you.

May 3   DASH to It!

If you live to age 55 or longer, you'll likely develop high blood pressure (hypertension). Even if your blood pressure ranges from 120/80 to 139/89 (prehypertension) you need to be cautious. Because the symptoms are silent, many people don't even know they have it. Why be concerned? Untreated, hypertension can lead to a heart attack or a stroke. That said, you probably can prevent (or at least postpone) hypertension by what you eat and do—starting now.

The DASH approach (Dietary Approaches to Stop Hypertension) works! It can lower your blood pressure (or risk for it), and likely reduce your blood cholesterol and weight, too, by eating:

- *Plenty of plant-based foods*—eight to ten fruit and vegetable servings and six to eight servings of grain products daily.
- *Enough low-fat or fat-free dairy foods*—two to three servings daily. Their calcium, magnesium, and potassium help control blood pressure.
- *Enough protein-rich foods*—four to five weekly servings of nuts and beans; no more than two daily servings of lean meat, poultry, or fish.

The benefit is greater with less sodium (down to 1,500 milligrams daily). (See January 16 for serving sizes.)

DASH to health during May, National High Blood Pressure Month.

- *Click the DASH eating plan:* Go to www.nhlbi.nih.gov/health/public/heart/hbp/dash. Start taking steps to follow it.
- *Eat food with less salt*—especially important if you're sodium sensitive. (Less than 2,400 milligrams daily.)
- *Put more "dash" in your lifestyle.* Try to fit 60 minutes of moderate activity into your day; 10 minutes at a time is okay. Work up a light sweat at least three times weekly.

May 4   Here's the Beef

Unless you're vegetarian, you probably eat beef and give little thought to its many health benefits. Because May is Beef Month, here's a beef brief.

Beef keeps good nutrition company. For less than 200 calories, a 3-ounce lean beef serving offers plenty of nutrition. Consider the Daily Values: *protein* (50%), *zinc* (39%), *vitamin B$_{12}$* (37%), *niacin* (a B vitamin) (18%), *vitamin B$_6$* (16%), and *iron* (14%). Nutrition brush-up: Zinc is needed for cell growth and repair, immunity, and hormone action; B vitamins, for releasing food's energy; and iron, for taking oxygen to cells, including muscles, to make energy.

There's more. Beef has two unique fatty acids: *conjugated linoleic acid* (CLA), perhaps with cancer-fighting qualities; and *stearic acid,* a saturated fat that doesn't act like one, with no effect on blood cholesterol, perhaps even lowering it.

Make a quick beef dish today. Start by buying lean meat (round and loin cuts); keep portions sensible (size of a deck of cards, about half of what you need daily) for less fat, saturated fat, and cholesterol.

- *Cook low-fat and quick.* Cut lean boneless sirloin in thin strips to stir-fry with vegetables.
- *Buy heat-and-eat.* Reheat a fully cooked boneless pot roast, and serve with veggies and rice, pasta, or whole-grain bread. Save leftovers for tomorrow's sandwiches.
- *Make a salad tonight.* Toss a hearty chef's salad, topped with strips of lean deli beef.

May 5   Passport to Health—Eating Mexican Style

Olé! Celebrate Mexican independence day with Mexican food or its Tex-Mex cousin, two of America's most popular ethnic cuisines.

Mexican menus deliver nutrition benefits from some common ingredients. Meat and poultry portions are sensible in size—providing enough, but not excessive, protein. Beans not only supply protein; they're iron- and fiber-rich, too. Tomato salsas are loaded with certain vitamins and antioxidants: beta carotene, vitamin C, and lycopene. Cheese (even low-fat) provides bone-building calcium. Tortillas, beans, and rice offer complex carbs; just go easy on preparation methods that add fat.

Celebrate with a new take on the always-popular taco.

- *Switch to soft.* Wrapped, folded, or flat, use soft tortillas (perhaps chipotle-flavored) with less fat than crispy ones, which may be fried.
- *Experiment with fillings.* Try broiled fish or shrimp with a lime squeeze, tomato, onion, and cilantro or a fruit salsa, *or* grilled chicken (asada) and salsa verde (green), *or* Mexican beans and rice, chili peppers, and picante sauce.
- *Take it easy* with guacamole, refried beans (made with lard), Cheddar and other cheeses, and sour cream.
- *Try a dessert taco:* chopped mango or papaya, mint, and flavored yogurt in a soft, warm tortilla.

Pineapple-Jalapeño Salsa

1 8-ounce can crushed pineapple in juice, undrained	1 canned pickled jalapeño pepper, minced (about 1 tablespoon)
⅓ cup chopped red onion	1 tablespoon lime juice
3 tablespoons chopped fresh cilantro	

In small bowl, combine all ingredients. Let stand 15 minutes, or cover and refrigerate up to 6 hours before using. Makes 6 servings.

Source: Canned Food Alliance

May 6 Got the Late-Night Munchies?

Do you take a snack break with each commercial break in the nightly news? Do you need a sweet before bedtime?

If you eat dinner early, maybe you really are hungry. A small snack to curb hunger is okay. Contrary to urban myths, late-evening calories are no more likely to promote weight gain and won't wake you up if you're sleepy. The real problems with late-night eating are lack of self-control and being out of touch with hunger cues. You may nibble out of habit, not hunger—especially when you stay up too late. That may lead to impulsive overeating—maybe high-fat or sugary snacks.

Strategize to avoid the late-night lure of food.

- *Pay attention.* Do hunger cues—or habit, boredom, or anxiety—trigger snacking? Take control.

- *Eat dinner somewhat later,* perhaps at 7 P.M. rather than 6 P.M. Or save dessert for later.
- *Go to bed earlier.* Eight hours of sleep gives you a mental edge to help control emotional eating any time of day.

May 7   Give the Gift of Health

Giving a gift for Mother's Day, a birthday, or no special occasion? Take a moment today to recognize a friend or family member, someone who stuck to a New Year's exercise resolution, met a work goal, or simply needs to know you care.

From your kitchen to theirs:

- *Share a pick-your-own outing.* Pack a decorative basket with farm-fresh berries, tree fruit, or garden vegetables. Tuck in your favorite recipe.
- *Wrap up a book.* Present a unique, health-focused cookbook, perhaps on ethnic cuisine, fruits and veggies, whole grains, grilling, or vegetarian dishes. Or pick a reliable consumer nutrition book, authored by a registered dietitian.
- *Present an ethnic food basket.* Go Italian with flavored pasta, sun-dried tomatoes, pasta sauce, a Parmesan cheese wedge, and a red-and-white checkered tablecloth. What could you tuck into an Asian- or a Mexican-inspired food basket?

May 8   Eggs-iting and Easy

Want a quick, inexpensive dinner? Try eggs—they're a protein bargain! A single egg counts as one of the 5 to 7 ounces of meat or meat alternate recommended daily.

Whole eggs offer more than protein: vitamins A and D, B vitamins, and phosphorus as well as some iron. (Eaten with vitamin C–rich fruit such as citrus, eggs' iron is absorbed better.) Egg yolk also contains lutein—good for healthy vision. For most healthy people, an egg a day is okay if their overall cholesterol intake stays under 300 milligrams daily. An egg has about 215 milligrams of cholesterol.

During May, National Egg Month, make an eggs-tra easy dish:

Stracciatella Florentine

2 14½-ounce cans fat-free, reduced-sodium chicken broth	4 eggs, well beaten
1 10-ounce package frozen chopped spinach	¼ cup grated Parmesan cheese
⅛ teaspoon ground nutmeg	1 cup cheese-and-garlic-flavored croutons, optional

In a large saucepan over high heat, bring broth to boiling. Add spinach. Cook until thawed, stirring occasionally with a fork to separate. Stir in nutmeg. Reduce heat to simmering. While stirring soup, slowly pour in eggs. (The eggs will set quickly in the simmering liquid.) Immediately remove from heat. Pour or ladle about 1 cup soup into each of six 10-ounce bowls. Sprinkle each with cheese and croutons, if desired. Makes 6 servings.

Source: American Egg Board

May 9   🖉 Sorting It Out!

Based on what you've heard or read, should you avoid some foods entirely? Almost 60 percent of consumers have that misconception, according to a recent survey. Some say, "We hear more about what we *can't* eat than what we *can*." Confused?

Sorting through the never-ending flow of nutrition information and misinformation isn't easy, especially when you're trying to make the best food choices for the whole family.

Before you let health and nutrition news make you feel like throwing all caution—and wisdom—to the wind:

- *Take the long view.* Make your food decisions on studies (plural!) from credible sources.
- *Listen to real experts.* Call a nutrition expert—perhaps in a university Extension office, hospital, or public health agency—where you live. Get a referral to a local registered dietitian at www.eatright.org.
- *Get up close and personal.* Make sure "hot" news in health applies to your personal needs. If you're not sure, talk it over with your doctor or a registered dietitian.

May 10   A "Slow-Mo" Workout

Need to tone your muscles? Improve your balance, flexibility, or posture? Relieve stress? Try Tai Chi. You don't need special shoes, clothes, or equipment—just a good instructor.

No matter what your age, the controlled dancelike movements of this centuries-old Chinese martial art can give you a good workout. In fact, its slow motion and gentle pace are the keys. As you move from one posture to another, you must concentrate, balance your shifting weight, relax your muscles, and control your breathing. Tip: since Tai Chi probably won't give you a real cardiovascular workout, fit walking, swimming, or other aerobic activity into your fitness plan, too.

Today, find out more about Tai Chi to see if you want to try it.

- *Check out a Tai Chi video.* Use it as your introduction.
- *Find a local Tai Chi class* at a health club, adult education program, or your hospital's community program. In the long run, you're best off with an instructor.

May 11   Do a Salad Makeover

Tired of the same old garden salad for dinner? National Salad Month is the perfect time for a salad makeover. A variety of vegetables and fruits add different nutrients, health-promoting phytonutrients, flavor, and appeal to your meals.

Salad making has no rules except: Use high-quality ingredients, clean fresh ingredients, and toss (if it's a garden salad) just before serving. Go easy with high-fat dressing.

Add more health-promoting benefits—and interest—to your salad today.

- *Mix your greens:* spinach, Romaine, red leaf, watercress. The deeper the color, the more carotenoids and health-promoting benefits.
- *Brighten with color:* tomato, broccoli florets, shredded carrots, green or red pepper, beets, even edible flowers.

- *Sweeten up:* mandarin orange segments, sliced strawberries, chopped apples, dried fruit.
- *Make it heartier:* sliced or chopped low-fat cheese, lean meat or turkey, tuna, shrimp, tofu, canned legumes (rinsed and drained), cooked pasta, rice, or bulgur.
- *Add crunch:* croutons, almonds, pecans, pistachios, pine nuts, walnuts, peanuts, sunflower seeds.
- *Herb it:* tarragon, chives, parsley, cilantro, marjoram, even mint.
- *Dress light, dress well:* spoon on just one or two tablespoons, not a ladleful of dressing.

May 12   In Case of Emergencies, Stock Up

Remember the Boy Scout motto? Be prepared! That's good advice for your pantry—in case a storm or an accident shuts off power.

If your power *does* go out, keep your refrigerator and freezer closed. Your refrigerator will stay cold for at least four to six hours; your freezer, about two days if it's full.

Before summer storm season hits, plan for unexpected emergencies.

- *Keep a three-day supply.* Get foods that keep in the cabinet: dry foods (nuts, trail mix, cereal, peanut butter); canned foods; foods in plastic bottles (jars can break); single-serve foods (you can't refrigerate leftovers); formula for babies; pet food. Keep needed medication, too. Remember a manual can opener.
- *Stock water.* Store enough for three days: 1 gallon per person per day. Buy bottled water in plastic containers. Or store your own in clean food-quality containers such as 2-liter soda bottles (not milk jugs). Unless your water comes from a well or untreated water supply, tap water doesn't need extra treatment.
- *Rotate your pantry.* If you've stocked up already, keep it fresh. Rotate every year or so.

May 13   Ladies' Turn

What makes women's nutrition needs unique? Perhaps less food energy (calories) to support a smaller body frame than men have and certainly the physiology of childbearing. Women: That said, keep this nutrition advice in mind:

- *During your childbearing years,* consume enough folate (400 micrograms daily) to protect against birth defects, enough calcium (1,000 milligrams daily) to help maintain healthy bones, enough iron (18 milligrams daily) to replace menstrual losses.
- *During and after your menopausal years,* consume enough calcium (1,200 to 1,500 milligrams daily) and more vitamin D (10 micrograms daily) to reduce bone loss with menopause, enough folate (400 micrograms daily) for protection from heart disease (like men, women are at high risk).

Another women's nutrition tip: soy foods, with their phytoestrogens (isoflavones), may help relieve the discomforts of premenstrual syndrome and menopause, and may help protect against breast cancer and bone loss after menopause. For more on soy foods, see April 2.

Women: During National Women's Health Week, commit to your best health.

- *For enough calcium:* low-fat milk, yogurt, calcium-fortified soy beverage, cheese, tofu processed with calcium sulfate, canned salmon with edible bones, kale, broccoli, calcium-fortified foods such as orange juice
- *For enough folate:* fortified grain foods, spinach, navy beans, peas, nuts, lentils, oranges
- *For enough iron:* meat, poultry, legumes, fortified breakfast cereal, enriched grain products, soybeans—plus vitamin C–rich foods for better iron absorption from plant-based foods

May 14   Whole in One

What comes to mind when you think of whole grains? Fiber? A single whole-grain food provides a whole array of health benefits.

Today's research is exploring how whole grains, eaten regularly in higher amounts, may offer these benefits: (1) reduce the chances of type 2 diabetes or at least help manage it by improving insulin's action; (2) lower total and LDL- (bad) cholesterol; (3) help protect you from some cancers, especially colorectal cancer, since fiber helps "sweep" your intestine; and (4) help with weight control, since high-fiber foods help you feel full longer after eating.

For the "whole" benefit, make at least three of your day's grain-product servings whole grain: whole-grain breads, brown rice, bulgur wheat, whole-grain barley, or hominy.

Tabouli

1 cup dry bulgur	*Dressing*
2 cups boiling water	⅓ cup vegetable or olive oil
3 tomatoes, seeded and chopped	⅓ cup lemon juice
1 bunch green onions, chopped	1 teaspoon salt
1 green pepper, chopped	½ teaspoon pepper
1 cucumber, diced	
1 bunch parsley, chopped (about 1 cup	
¼ cup chopped mint, optional	

Add bulgur to water; cover and let stand 30 minutes. Drain away any remaining liquid. Mix vegetables and herbs with bulgur. For dressing, combine oil, lemon juice, salt, and pepper; combine with the bulgur mixture. Refrigerate at least 2 hours before serving. Serves 8.

Adapted from: Wheat Foods Council

May 15 Sneak 'Em In

Have a challenge getting your family to eat vegetables? Is your family well intentioned, but poor at meal planning? Do they simply resist or dislike veggies?

Then maybe you need to get sneaky. Your family deserves the chance to experience new flavors, get the health benefits, and ultimately learn to enjoy vegetables in new ways.

If veggies meet with family resistance:

• *Serve salsa.* Salsa (with tomatoes, beans, or other veggies) served with pita, bagel, or tortilla chips doesn't seem like a vegetable.
• *Blend them in.* Put shredded carrots in mashed potatoes, or mix them with potatoes for twice-baked potatoes, chopped broccoli

in macaroni and cheese, layered zucchini in lasagna, or shredded spinach in slaw.

- *Wrap it up.* Hide veggies in a tortilla wrap, under pizza cheese, or at the bottom of a pita.
- *Serve one-dish meals.* That way, they can't push away the veggie side dish.

May 16   Cook Savvy—Kick It Up a Notch

Think you need to give up flavor for nutrition, or that healthful foods just don't taste as good? An astounding number of people do. And they give up on smart eating as a result. Fact is, good taste and good nutrition can go together!

For the best flavor, start with quality ingredients at their peak. Store them properly; use them while they're still fresh and safe to eat. Avoid overcooking. And serve foods at their right temperature: milk and salads cold, hot meals hot.

Today, kick up the flavor in nutrient-rich foods.

- *Juice the rice.* Instead of water, cook rice in tomato juice or broth.
- *Grill or roast your veggies* to give a sweet, smoky flavor.
- *Add spark with sharp cheese.* Try just a *little* feta, blue, Parmesan, or sharp Cheddar on salads or vegetables.
- *Concentrate the stock.* Simmering to reduce the juices from cooking meat, poultry, and fish makes a nice glaze—and flavorful alternative to gravy.

May 17   De-Vine—The Benefits of Wine

Red or white? The time-honored rule—white wine with chicken or fish, red with meat—doesn't take into account a meal's layers of flavors or the distinctive flavor differences among red and white wines. Some wine experts say the right wine is a matter of personal taste anyway. After all, each person perceives flavor differently.

Drinking wine—either white or red—in moderate amounts may offer some heart-healthy benefits, perhaps boosting HDL- (good) cholesterol, helping prevent LDL- (bad) cholesterol from forming, or helping prevent blood platelets that cause heart attacks and strokes from clotting. Plant substances in grapes, such as resveratrol (flavonoid) and tannins, may contribute to these benefits. The alcohol may be a factor, too.

To get heart-healthy benefits from the vine:

- *Enjoy the wine you like,* but no more than one 5-ounce glass of wine daily for women; for men, it's two.
- *Drink grape juice.* If you don't drink wine, grape juice may offer some of the same heart-healthy benefits.

May 18   Bone Up with Impact-ivities

Does your fitness regimen help keep your bones healthy? Probably so, *if* your regular physical activities are weight-bearing and *if* you consume enough calcium and vitamin D.

Like muscles, your bones need a workout to stay strong. What's weight-bearing? Any activity that requires your feet and legs to carry your weight. Walking, jogging, stair stepping, dancing, playing volleyball or tennis, even mowing the grass or shoveling snow are; swimming and cycling aren't. Resistance activities, such as weight lifting, promote bone health, too.

Put a little more weight on your bones.

- *Walk up, walk down some stairs.* Start with a flight or two, then gradually do more during the week. Steer clear of the elevator.
- *Lift weights as you phone chat.* Just grab some canned foods, milk jugs, or whatever else is handy, and lift!
- *Carry your grocery bags.* Forget the shopping cart if you're not buying too much.

May 19   Give Your "Self" a Makeover

Very few women can ever achieve the fashion model "ideal body," no matter what their approach. So why set yourself up for failure, guilt, and frustration with an unrealistic and perhaps unhealthy weight goal?

Whether you're male or female, focus your mind-set and your weight strategies on being fit and healthy.

- *Accept yourself.* Remember, healthy bodies come in different shapes and sizes. Set your goals on what's right for you.
- *Remind yourself.* You don't need to buy into the often unattainable, unhealthy "sleek" standard. Magazine pictures are likely "improved" anyway.
- *Care for yourself.* Dump the stress of misguided goals. Eat smart and move more to be your personal best.

If you think you need a makeover:

- *Set a smart weight goal,* one that's just right for you. Check with your physician. If you're overweight, losing just 10 pounds can make a health difference if your cholesterol, blood pressure, or blood sugar level is too high.
- *Take one step this week* to be more fit and healthy. Keep it up!

May 20   Creeping Calories

The average American consumed about 340 more calories a day in the late 1990s than in the mid-1980s, and at least 500 more calories daily since the 1950s. At the same time, Americans are less physically active. How about you?

How much food energy (calories) is enough, but not too much? Among other things, the right amount for you depends on your age, gender, and how much you move. To lose a pound, you need to consume 3,500 calories less than you consume. Do that by consuming less, moving more, or both. Here's daily calorie advice for the "average adult."

	Women	Men
If you're sedentary, like most people	1,600 calories	2,200 calories
If you're physically active	2,200 calories	2,800 calories

(Source: Dietary Guidelines for Americans, 2000)

Take a few minutes today for a reality check. Count your calories.

- *From food labels:* Jot down the amount in your portions. Are they bigger than a label serving? Be honest with yourself. Remember snacks and drinks.
- *Ask for calorie info in restaurants.* Many fast-food places have it.
- *Buy a pocket calorie counter.* Or check calories in food online at www.nal.usda.gov/fnic/foodcomp.
- *Add them up.* Surprised?

May 21   Tofu—For You?

Tofu—you know it's healthful. In fact, this cheeselike soy food supplies heart-healthy soy protein and B vitamins. If made with calcium salt, it can be high in calcium, yet low in sodium. Fat content varies, so check labels.

So, what kind do you buy? Easy: *firm* for grilling and stir-fries; *soft* for puréeing, mashing, and mixing in meatloaf; and *silken* for the smoothest texture in dips, dressings, puddings, smoothies, and sauces.

Store it unopened in the fridge. Exception: Tofu in aseptic packaging doesn't need refrigeration until it's opened. After opening, refrigerate tofu in water, change the water daily, and use it within a week. If tofu smells sour, toss it.

Ready to prepare tofu? First rinse and drain it. Mild-flavored tofu soaks up the great flavors of other ingredients.

Prepare an easy tofu dish with puréed soft tofu in place of cream, cream cheese, sour cream, or mayonnaise.

Easy To-fredo Sauce

8 ounces fettuccini pasta
12 ounces silken tofu, drained
⅓ cup Parmigiano-Reggiano cheese, grated
2 tablespoons soybean oil

1 tablespoon soymilk, plain
¾ teaspoon fresh garlic, minced
½ teaspoon white pepper, ground
¼ teaspoon salt

Prepare pasta as directed on package; drain and set aside. Place remaining ingredients in food processor or blender. Purée 1 to 2 minutes until smooth; add 1 to 2 tablespoons soymilk to thin, if desired. Microwave in a microwave-safe bowl on high 2 to 3 minutes until warm, stirring occasionally, or heat in small saucepan on stovetop over medium-high heat 3 to 4 minutes until warm, stirring constantly. Do not overheat. Serve immediately over hot pasta. Makes 4 servings.

Pesto Sauce Variation: Purée 1 tablespoon chopped fresh basil and 2 teaspoons chopped fresh oregano with the tofu.

Source: United Soybean Board

May 22   Stress Busters

Ever feel like you have it all the stress you can handle, perhaps even more? Soft music or aromatherapy might offer relief for a while, but regular physical activity may give more stress-relieving benefits over the long haul.

Why? The reasons aren't fully understood. Several factors may come into play: (1) feelings of relaxation and euphoria, as many neurotransmitters, including endorphins, get involved; (2) less nervous tension as muscles relax; (3) more self-worth as you control your body; and (4) better eating since physically active people tend to eat healthier. Well nourished, you'll handle stress better, too.

Reduce emotional stress during National Mental Health Month by moving more.

- *Skip tension-producing activities,* such as competitive sports or crowded workout classes or gyms, if they stress you.
- *Pick what works for you:* yoga, Tai Chi, or Pilates that help relax your mind; brisk walking or other aerobic activities that help with stress control; or tennis, racquetball, or other vigorous sports that release adrenaline.
- *Do it—even when you're stressed!* A 10-minute physical activity break (walking, stretching, climbing stairs) every 90 minutes may be just what you need.

May 23   Be Good to Your Joints

Experience ongoing joint pain, stiffness, or swelling for longer than two weeks? See your doctor. You may have arthritis; one in three American adults do. The sooner you get an accurate diagnosis (there are more than a hundred forms) and treatment, the less pain and joint damage. *Caution:* Despite the allure of dietary supplements, talk to your physician before taking any to treat arthritis. Scientific evidence is still lacking on their effectiveness; some may interfere with medication.

May is National Arthritis Month, a good time to take stock of how you protect against the risk or progression of this debilitating disease.

- *Commit to a healthy weight.* Drop a few pounds if you're overweight. Extra weight adds extra stress to hips and knees.
- *Reach for citrus.* According to new research, its vitamin C may be among the antioxidants that reduce osteoarthritis risk and its progression.
- *Eat smart overall.* Science hasn't yet uncovered clear links between nutrition and arthritis. But smart eating certainly won't hurt!
- *Get moving.* If you already have arthritis, ask your doctor for the right range-of-motion and strengthening exercises. Try walking or aquatic exercise; neither jars your joints. Physical activity actually helps reduce pain and can increase range of movement.
- *Stretch.* Proper stretching after warming up helps your joints and muscles stay flexible.

May 24   Why Diets Don't Stick

Did dieting ever do you in? Truth is, most "diets" don't work—at least not for long. Too soon, you've cheated. You're off your diet, even gained back what you lost, and then some. Why does dieting so often fail?

- *Giving up too much.* It's hard to resist a "forbidden" food. Restricting calories so much that you feel hungry is a recipe for failure.
- *Missing out on motion.* You lose weight easier and keep it off better if you move more, too.
- *Overlooking the big picture.* Quick fixes rarely focus on the only real solution: lifestyle changes.

Rethink your notion of dieting today, unless guided by your health care professional.

- *Get real.* Set a realistic goal, matched to your lifestyle. Write it down.
- *Plan to go slowly.* Losing a half to one pound weekly is healthy and more sustainable.
- *Ease stress.* Too much stress often leads to emotional overeating and cheating.
- *Fit it in.* Eat a variety of nutrient-rich foods with fewer total calories than you'd normally eat. Just follow healthful eating advice. That might mean smaller portions. And fit in more motion!

May 25   Grill Safe

What's on your Memorial Day menu? Chances are, you're opening the summer season with a barbecue. To keep your meal perfect, keep it safe!

Your grilled meal can be an ideal medium for bacteria to multiply—fast! A potential result? Food-borne illness for you, your family, and your guests.

To keep harmful bacteria at bay whenever you grill:

- *Marinate in the fridge, not on the countertop.* Set aside any unused marinade for basting. Toss out leftover marinade used with raw meat, poultry, or fish—unless you heat it to a rolling boil first.
- *Clean the grill.* Get rid of debris from the last cookout.
- *Precook wisely.* If you partly cook food in your kitchen first, grill it right away. Or thoroughly cook it ahead, refrigerate, and just reheat it on the grill.
- *Cook thoroughly on both sides.* Use a meat thermometer to check for safety and doneness: burgers, 160°F; poultry breasts, 170°F; steaks, 145° to 170°F; pork, 160°F.
- *Transfer cooked foods to clean plates with clean utensils.* Keep raw meat, poultry, and seafood juices away from cooked foods, vegetables, and fruits.
- *Serve right away!* In hot weather, the keeping time is an hour or less.

May 26 🏃 Get Fit with a Friend

Need motivation to stay active? Perhaps you savor solitary workouts. Or maybe social interaction with a fitness partner is a better success strategy.

Interestingly, companionship often increases the odds of sticking with a fitness program. After all, someone's waiting for you—and moving with you. A partner can support your fitness efforts; you're there to reciprocate. Keeping up with someone else may add to the challenge. What's more, being together can make physical activity a lot more fun and social. And you can keep moving while you talk.

It's National Physical Fitness and Sports Month. Begin your fitness partnership today.

- *Find a companion:* your spouse, another family member, a neighbor, or a friend.
- *Find an organized sport or activity* wherever people gather for active fun, perhaps a fitness or community center, track, or cycling club.
- *Sign up for a fun run or group bike ride.* Training together for the big day will keep you on track.

May 27 🍎 Time for an Oil Change

Ever think of olives as a fruit? Not sweet, but rich in healthful fats, olives are more than a savory ingredient and finger food.

Why so healthful? Compared with vegetable oils, olive oil has far more *monounsaturated fat* (the good kind). And it has little saturated fat. That's the key—"monos" may lower total and LDL- (bad) cholesterol in blood and perhaps raise HDL- (good) cholesterol, while saturated fats raise both total and LDL-cholesterol. (The risk for heart disease goes up when total and LDL levels are higher and/or HDLs are lower.) Because it comes from plants, olive oil has no cholesterol.

Before you "chug" a jigger of olive oil, remember: It's not calorie free. A tablespoon of olive oil has 14 fat grams and 120 calories, slightly more than the same amount of butter or margarine.

For flavor and health benefits, toss salads with olive-oil vinaigrette.

South American Garbanzo Salad

2 cups canned garbanzo beans, drained and rinsed
⅔ cup California black ripe olives, cut into wedges
½ cup diced red bell pepper
⅓ cup sliced green onion

¼ cup chopped cilantro
2 tablespoons extra-virgin olive oil
1½ tablespoons sherry vinegar
1 hard-cooked egg, finely diced
Salt and pepper to taste

In a large mixing bowl, combine garbanzo beans, olives, red bell pepper, green onion, and cilantro. Mix in oil and vinegar, then gently toss in egg. Season with salt and pepper, and serve at room temperature. Makes 4 servings.
Source: California Olive Industry

May 28 Bone Up for Health

It's a fact of adult aging that more years mean less bone. Keeping bones dense and out of the "fracture zone" depends on three things: (1) your starting bone mass; (2) your habits that slow bone loss; and (3) osteoporosis risks you can't control.

Anyone past age 65 is at risk for osteoporosis. Your risk goes up—even sooner—if any of these describe you: family history of fractures or osteoporosis, female, Caucasian or Asian, underweight or small-framed, early menopause, chronic low calcium intake, smoker, inactive, heavy drinker of alcoholic beverages. High doses of thyroid medication or prolonged use of cortisone medications increase the risk, too. Although women's risk is higher, 20 percent of hip fractures happen in men.

During May, Osteoporosis Prevention Month and beyond, bone up!

- *Cut your calcium deficit.* Eat enough calcium-rich foods to hit the guideline: 1,000 milligrams daily for adults to age 50; 1,200 milligrams daily after that.
- *Get enough vitamin D.* It helps your body absorb calcium efficiently. Most milk has it. Take a supplement with vitamin D if you get calcium elsewhere.
- *Exercise for bone health.* Weight-bearing activity, done standing up, builds bones.
- *Schedule a bone density scan* if you're high risk.

May 29 🛒 Enough's Enough

You've seen restaurant menus featuring deluxe burgers with 8-ounce patties, hefty 12-ounce steaks, half a roasted chicken. That's more food than you need. Five to 7 ounces of meat a day is enough for most people. You might enjoy it in two to three servings or in one bigger portion.

How much meat, poultry, or fish constitutes a food-group serving? Visualize a deck of cards. That's the size of one food-group serving of cooked of boneless, lean meat, poultry, or fish—3 to 4 ounces.

Use this buying guide to help you shop right.

Number of 3-Ounce Servings (Cooked) per Pound of Uncooked Food

Food	Servings
Meat	
No bone: ground or boneless meat	4
Some bone: steaks, roast, chops	2 to 3
A lot of bone: short ribs, shoulder cuts	1 to 2
Poultry	
Whole chicken	2
Boneless chicken breast	4
Whole turkey	2
Boneless turkey roast	3
Ground turkey	4
Fish	
Whole	1⅓ to 1½
Fillets	3⅓ to 4
Steaks without bone	3
Scallops, cooked lobster or crabmeat	4
Shrimp, headless, unpeeled	3
Shrimp, peeled and deveined	4

May 30 🌾 Energy Booster, or Not?

More energy, less stress: we all want it, but what really works and what doesn't?

First, what *doesn't*. Supplements might purport to help you cope with stress or boost your energy. But emotional stress doesn't increase nutrient needs. And vitamin pills won't cause your body cells to produce extra energy or more brain power. Only smart eating does that.

So-called energy drinks often "power-up" their marketing with carbs, high caffeine, even ephedrine as the ingredient behind the claims. Yet high-carb drinks or energy bars won't fuel body cells right away. Caffeine only gives a short-term energy boost. And the stimulant ephedrine can be dangerous (it's been linked to having a heart attack, a stroke, tremors, even death).

Now what does work: consistently eating a variety of foods; drinking enough fluids (dehydration causes fatigue); being regularly physically active (stamina booster); learning to relieve stress and to sleep enough.

Boost your energy today effectively.

- *Drink enough fluids:* about 8 cups a day, more if you perspire a lot.
- *Eat regular meals with a variety of foods.* Meal skipping causes energy dips.
- *Take time to be more active.* Make it an ongoing habit.

May 31   Soft Drinks, Hard Facts

Thirsty? Do you reach for a soft drink? If so, how big are your gulps? Fifty years ago, a 6-ounce bottle (75 calories) was the norm. Today 20-ounce (250 calories) plastic bottles often tumble from vending machines. And convenience stores pour up to 64 ounces (800 calories) per big cup! Now add 'em up: how many soda calories do you drink in a day? Most adults need just 1,600 to 2,400 calories a day from *all* their food and drinks.

Regular or diet, sodas are okay now and then. But as an everyday drink choice, do they crowd out nutrient-rich drinks like milk? Regular sodas deliver sugars (carbs), but essentially no other nutrients. Consumed in place of a calcium-rich option, they may contribute to bone loss. Sugary sodas contribute to tooth decay, but no more than juice or other carbohydrate-rich foods.

To take the now-and-then soft drink approach:

- *Order the small size,* even if "bigger" seems like a better value.
- *Pour less.* If a 20-ounce or bigger bottle is your only choice, pour a smaller amount in a cup and save the rest.
- *Decide when*—but not all the time for sodas.
- *Switch* to flavored milk for a more healthful option.

June 1   Milk It—For All It's Worth

Penny for penny, drinking milk's the most cost-effective way to consume bone-building calcium—more so than calcium-fortified juice, soy milk, breakfast bars, and other calcium-fortified foods. (See August 8 for more about calcium.)

And milk offers you more: for just one cup of fat-free, low-fat, or whole milk you not only get 30% Daily Value (DV) for calcium, you also get 20% DV or more for vitamin D, riboflavin, and phosphorus; and 10% DV or more for protein, vitamin B_{12}, potassium, niacin, and vitamin A.

During June, National Dairy Month, and beyond, enjoy milk: in your morning coffee or tea, as an afternoon snack drink (strawberry, banana, or other flavored milk), or in a new-to-you dairy-rich recipe. (*Hint:* Drink your cereal milk, too.)

Mango Yogurt Soup

1 pound ripe mangoes, peeled, seeded, and cut in pieces	⅛ teaspoon nutmeg, fresh grated or ground
1 cup low-fat plain yogurt	Sprig of parsley or mint, edible
1 cup milk	flowers, or thin slices of lime, for
¼ cup sugar	garnish
⅛ teaspoon cinnamon	

In a blender or food processor, purée mango with yogurt, milk, sugar, cinnamon, and nutmeg to desired smoothness. For thinner soup, add more milk to taste. Chill and serve as a cold soup. For dessert, add less milk for a thicker, richer-tasting puddinglike consistency. Makes 4 servings.

Source: Produce for Better Health Foundation

June 2 🏃 Life's a Beach

Have you planned your summer getaways yet? Relaxing on the beach with a good book is great, but this year put plenty of *active* leisure fun in your vacation plans, too.

- *Gather active beach or water gear.* Get out the Frisbees, beach tennis or badminton equipment, beach balls, a kite, masks and snorkels—whatever gets you moving on or near the water.
- *Go dude!* Enjoy active relaxation at a western dude ranch, a family camp, or a park campground. Take your hiking boots.
- *Plan ahead for balance.* Visiting a theme park? Fit in a day or two for water play, biking, or some other active fun, too. In the city, take a walking tour.
- *Pack walking or running shoes.* Make time for daily walks on the beach, around the city, on the trail or ship's deck, or in any place your summer vacation takes you.

June 3 ✍ Come Clean

When fruits and vegetables are summer fresh, do you need to wash them, even if you peel away the skin and only eat the insides? Yes!

Washing removes debris and residues from the outside surfaces and crevices of produce. Cutting through unwashed produce can carry dirt or bacteria to the inside flesh.

To clean your fresh produce any time of year:

- *Choose produce carefully.* Reject any with decay, mold, insect holes, or surface cuts. Remove bruised or damaged spots that may harbor bacteria or mold.
- *Use separate cutting boards*—one for cleaning produce, another for raw meat, poultry, and fish. Color code the boards, or label them with a permanent marker. Use plastic boards; wooden cutting boards can harbor bacteria.
- *Remove outer leaves* on lettuce, cabbage, and other leafy vegetables. "Rust" spots on lettuce aren't harmful.

- *Wash produce with clean, running water just before eating.* Unless made for cleaning produce, skip soap; it leaves residue. You don't need a vegetable wash (made from baking soda and citric acid) either; if you do use it, rinse well.
- *Scrub firm produce with a vegetable brush:* melons, cucumbers, carrots, foods with edible peels.
- *Store cleaned produce in clean containers or plastic storage bags.*
- *Keep your refrigerator produce drawer clean.* Wash and sanitize it often.

June 4   🍎 Tea Time

Care for a refreshing glass of cold iced tea? Hot tea with your breakfast? Green tea to go with sushi or dim sum? Besides flavor and relaxation, tea drinking may offer health benefits.

Although the research isn't definitive, tea's *catechins* and other *polyphenols* may help reduce your risk for cancer, heart disease, and stroke by protecting your body cells from damage by free radicals, which are formed in nature and when your body uses oxygen to make energy. Here's the clincher: You may need 4 to 6 cups of tea (black, oolong, or green) daily for the benefits.

Smile about this: When brewed, tea leaves release *fluoride,* which helps tooth enamel stay strong. Tea also may help reduce plaque and inhibit cavity-forming bacteria.

Try these when you set your "tea time"—especially during June, National Iced Tea Month:

- *Hot or iced, order tea latte,* prepared like coffee latte—and get milk's calcium benefits, too.
- *As a summer refresher, make mint tea lemonade.* Steep green tea with fresh mint. Mix in spoonfuls of frozen lemonade concentrate to taste. Chill.
- *As a switch from sugar or honey,* sweeten tea with citrus slices, ginger, or a cinnamon stick.
- *Try chai:* spiced milk tea with origins in India, often made with cloves, cinnamon, nutmeg, cardamom, and pepper. Ice it down!

June 5 📝 Improvement, Not Perfection

Do you ever grab chips when you intended to go for carrots? Instead of feeling guilty or giving up, remember: Nobody's perfect. Improvement, not perfection, is a realistic, sensible, and far more effective goal.

Fact is, there's no such thing as a "perfect" way to eat or stay active. Your best approach is all about you!

Today work on a realistic mind-set to be better (not perfect): eat a little smarter or move a little more.

- *Remember, there are no rules, but instead guidelines*—to help you eat and do what's right for you and your health.
- *Cut yourself some slack.* If you slip up today, just get back to your healthful routine tomorrow without guilt. What counts is what you eat or do over several days, not just today.
- *Give yourself credit for improvement.* What's one way you've been eating smarter or moving more recently?

June 6 🌾 Skin Deep

Can good nutrition help aging skin? Perhaps a little.

Your skin is genetically programmed to age. The rate depends on your genes, as well as your lifestyle and health. With age, you lose some fat padding under your skin's epidermis (top layer), and skin cells replace themselves more slowly. Less collagen and connective tissue in your dermis (next layer down) means less skin elasticity (more wrinkles).

Good nutrition can help a little. Vitamin C, in many fruits and vegetables, helps form collagen in the skin and connective tissue. Zinc, from whole grains, meat, and legumes, is part of collagen-maintaining enzymes and helps keep cell membranes healthy. Protein, from legumes, fish, poultry, meat, and dairy foods, helps replace all cells, including skin cells. And antioxidants, in fruits and vegetables, may help protect your skin from some changes caused by aging and sunlight.

Slow skin aging with these tactics:

- *Protect your skin from sun.* Ultraviolet rays cause photoaging, which permanently damages the epidermis and the dermis (and increases skin cancer risk).
- *Moisturize your skin well.*
- *If you smoke, quit.*
- *Eat smart,* with enough food variety to provide the nutrients and the antioxidants that promote healthy skin.

June 7   Build a Better Burger

What's cooking on your grill? Chances are, burgers—at least for one meal or another.

How do you grill the perfect burger? You can't judge doneness by its color. The middle may be brown before your burger's fully cooked, especially if you mix a dark sauce into raw ground meat. *For safety's sake,* do away with guessing and use a meat thermometer or barbecue fork thermometer. Cooked properly, hamburgers and ground meat measure in at 160°F; ground poultry burgers, at 165°F.

For great, good-for-you burger flavor:

- *Mix in some herbs:* garlic, chives, and basil; oregano and chili powder; ginger and coriander; cilantro, pepper flakes, and onion. Easy on the salt.
- *Go lean.* Choose lean ground meat or poultry for patties. For something different, grill soyburgers or salmon patties.
- *Think beyond catsup, lettuce, and tomato.* Top your burger with chutney, barbecue sauce, or salsa; roasted peppers, spinach leaves, or watercress; havarti, provolone, or blue-veined cheese.
- *Switch from buns.* Try a tortilla wrap, foccacia, naan, a soft bagel, or a whole-wheat English muffin.

June 8   Aqua-Size for Fitness

Enjoy the pool? Cool! No doubt, the pool is a great place to de-stress your life. But swimming—or aquatic exercise—also can give you a great, low- or no-impact workout.

A 1-hour aquatic workout can be a calorie burner: up to 400 to 700 calories, depending on the intensity. It's great for strength training; the natural resistance of water exercise is twelve times that of moving in air. For cross training, frequent water exercise can help improve your walking, running, and spinning (pedaling). And many water activities improve both flexibility and range of motion.

If weight-bearing activities are painful or difficult for you, a water workout might be your answer. Because water supports your weight and reduces impact, aquatic exercise helps you strengthen and tone and improve your endurance without stressing your joints or back.

Ready to try? In the shallow water (chest or waist deep):

- *Water walk.* Stay erect, rather than leaning forward. Swing your arms and shoulders as you walk.
- *Twist*, with legs apart, feet flat, arms just above the water.
- *Water dance.* Hop, move your arms to the rhythm.
- *Sign up for an aquatic exercise class.* Check your community college or public pool for a class.

June 9   Basically Barley

Good in soups and stews, hearty and healthful, barley's got lots to offer.

Like other whole grains, barley supplies plenty of *complex carbs,* yet little fat. It's also a good fiber source—*soluble fiber* to help lower blood cholesterol levels and reduce heart disease risk, and *insoluble fiber* to help your intestine work normally and perhaps help reduce colorectal cancer risk. Barley's phytonutrients may have related benefits. Besides that, barley contains several *B vitamins, selenium, iron, magnesium,* and *zinc.*

Add pearl barley to tonight's dinner.

- *In meatballs.* Cook barley according to package instructions. Then mix it with raw ground meat and other ingredients before shaping and cooking.
- *In salad.* Cook first, then substitute barley in salads that use cooked pasta or rice.

Barley Apricot Pilaf

1¾ cups (14-ounce can) chicken broth	¼ cup chopped dried apricots
1 cup orange juice	¼ cup raisins
¼ cup white wine	½ cup toasted slivered almonds
1 cup pearl barley	1 teaspoon grated orange peel

Combine broth, juice, wine, barley, dried apricots, and raisins in a saucepan. Bring to a boil. Cover, reduce heat to low, and cook 45 minutes or until barley is tender and liquid is absorbed. Sprinkle pilaf with almonds and orange peel just before serving. Makes 6 servings.

Source: National Barley Foods Council

June 10 Veggie Good Ideas

A trivia question for June, National Fresh Fruit and Vegetable Month: What vegetables top the U.S. 10 best-seller list? (Potatoes, head lettuce, tomatoes, onions, carrots, celery, corn, broccoli, green cabbage, and cucumber) Now, reach beyond those to meet the day's goal for fruit and vegetable servings: five to nine a day. In the vegetable category, go for beets, red cabbage, sweet potatoes, red pepper. Or try something more extraordinary.

Commit to trying one new vegetable today.

* *In a tossed salad*
* *As a raw, finger-food snack*
* *In a quick stir-fry*

Try one of these specialty vegetables today:

* *Celeriac* (seh-LER-ee-ak), a sweet, celery-flavored root, tastes good raw or cooked.
* *Chayote* (cheye-OH-tay), mild in flavor, can be prepared like squash.
* *Fennel* looks like celery, tastes like anise. Slice the raw bulb and stalks; add to salads or enjoy with a dip. The leaves are great in salads, too.
* *Hearts of palm,* fresh or canned, blend nicely in salads. No cooking needed.
* *Kale,* a leafy vegetable, can be enjoyed raw or cooked, like spinach.

- *Kohlrabi* (KOHL-ra-bee) tastes like a turnip. Cook it in soup or stew, or enjoy it raw and crunchy.
- *Tomatillo* (tohm-ah-TEE-oh) looks like a small green tomato with a paperlike husk. It adds citruslike flavor to salad and salsa.

June 11   Kids in Your Kitchen

School's out! If you have kids at home—or if you want to enjoy time with a niece, a nephew, grandkids, or young friends—why not share kitchen time this summer?

Kitchen experiences teach kids all kinds of facts (about foods and science) and skills (measuring, counting, reading, following directions). Kitchen time helps develop self-confidence, independence, self-esteem ("I made it!"), curiosity, and responsibility.

All that—and cooking is a great way to share time together!

Today, plan fun kitchen time with kids.

- *Start with hand and table washing.*
- *Match tasks to the child's abilities.* Preschoolers can stir, pour, and shake, and, as they develop, spread, mix, and knead. With supervision, school-age kids also can measure, cut, and grate.
- *Show safety.* Teach young children to stay away from sharp objects and hot surfaces and utensils. Help older kids use appliances safely with supervision.
- *Try to teach just one skill at a time.*
- *Talk about* tastes, smells, textures, sounds, what they see.
- *Accept messes.* Kids don't have the coordination and skills that you have.
- *Make cleanup part of learning.* Cleanup is part of the messy, creative things we do.

June 12   Worth It?

Wonder if there's any truth to the suggestion that shark cartilage or lecithin may help prevent or cure disease? Here's what health experts say:

- *Lecithin and arthritis (or other health problems):* Your body makes lecithin. So taking more doesn't seem to offer any benefits. Synthetic lecithin isn't absorbed well, anyway.
- *Shark cartilage and cancer:* Limited research shows no role in blocking tumor formation. Any active substances in shark cartilage haven't been identified. And it might be risky for pregnant women, people with heart disease, and those who are recovering from surgery or wounds.

  Note: The U.S. Food and Drug Administration warns against the serious, even deadly, side effects of these supplements: aristolochic acid, chaparral, comfrey, ephedrine, germander, lobelia, magnolia-stephania preparation, willow bark, wormwood, yohimbe.

For your safety, check with your physician before trying a supplement. If you have an adverse reaction:

- *Tell your physician and pharmacist* about the supplement name, type, and your dosage. Keep the container so you can identify it.
- *Report serious problems* to the U.S. Food and Drug Administration (FDA) MedWatch hotline: (1-800-FDA-1088), fax (1-800-FDA-0178), or online www.fda.gov/medwatch/).
- *Contact your nearest FDA District Office* with your concern or complaint. Look in the government pages of the phone book.

June 13   Passport to Health—Eating Japanese Style

What comes to mind when you think of Japanese food? Rice, sushi, tofu, vegetables? An artfully presented tray of all those things?

Beyond beauty, Japanese eating is healthful eating. It's mostly low in fat and low in calories, with most food energy from carbohydrate-rich foods, such as rice and noodles. It features plenty of fish, with heart-healthy omega-3 fatty acids; soy foods, low-fat protein sources that also supply potentially cancer-protective isoflavones; nutrient-rich, phytonutrient-rich vegetables; and plenty of food variety.

Take a lesson today from the Japanese table.

- *Use chopsticks to help you eat more slowly.* You'll "hear" your hunger and fullness cues and enjoy food more.
- *Make it look good.* Eat from a nice plate. Include lots of vegetables for color, flavor, and nutrition. Garnish with herbs, fruit, or edible flowers.
- *Serve more fish, more veggies, and perhaps soy foods.* (See May 21 tips on tofu.)
- *Enjoy food and family table time*—one of several Japanese dietary guidelines.

June 14 🍎 Peachy Keen

Just peachy. Plum good. Top banana. Peaches 'n' cream. Think about it. In our everyday expressions, fruit connotes good things.

Peaches rank in consumers' "top fruit 10." Along with nectarines (very close cousin), a peach's yellow flesh contains antioxidants—*beta carotene, flavonoids,* and some *vitamin C*—which may protect against ongoing health problems, such as heart disease and cancer. White-fleshed peaches and nectarines supply potentially cancer-fighting *catechins.* And their skins supply both *fiber* and other phytonutrients.

For peachy-keen summer refreshment, enjoy cut-up peaches, nectarines, or any fruit with yogurt in an oversized waffle cone. Or try this:

Blushing Nectarine* Sangria

1 3-inch strip orange peel	½ cup orange juice
¼ cup sugar	¼ cup freshly squeezed lemon juice
3 ripe fresh nectarines or peaches	1 chilled 10-ounce bottle club soda
1 bottle white zinfandel (may substitute alcohol-free white zinfandel)	

In a large bowl, bruise orange peel with sugar to release oils. Pit and crush one nectarine; add to bowl with wine, stirring to blend. Let steep in refrigerator several hours or overnight. Strain into pitcher; stir in orange and lemon juices. Pit and slice remaining 2 nectarines, and add to pitcher. Pour in club soda just before serving. Serve over ice in large glasses. Makes 6 servings.

Source: California Tree Fruit Agreement

*May substitute peaches

June 15   Active? Drink Enough?

Imagine you've just had a great workout. You're really sweating! Are you drinking enough to stay well hydrated? Dehydration often starts with flushed skin, fatigue, increased body temperature, and faster breathing and pulse rates. From there, you might feel the early signs of heat exhaustion or heat stroke: dizziness, weakness, harder breathing.

To keep properly hydrated, drink plenty of water before, during, and after physical activity, even if you don't feel thirsty.

- *2 hours before:* 2 cups
- *15 minutes ahead:* 1 to 2 cups
- *Every 15 minutes while you're active:* ½ to 1 cup
- *After you're active:* 3 cups for each pound of weight you lose while you're active

To make sure you drink enough:

- *Carry a water bottle.* Or know where a water fountain or station is. (A medium mouthful is not much, just about 1 ounce; 8 ounces is a cup.)
- *Weigh yourself before and after a heavy workout.* That way you'll know how much fluid you need to replace.
- *Check your urine.* If it's light and clear (lemon juice color), you're likely drinking enough. If it's darker (apple juice color), you're dehydrated.

June 16   Locally Grown

Looking for a summer outing, something that's fun, educational, and good for you, too? Enjoy the "earthy experience" of a farmer's market and buy your produce directly from small, local growers.

Throughout the country, local markets and U-pick-it farms are "cropping" up with seasonal produce, grown almost in your back-yard. Here's what makes them fun:

- *Unique, regional produce*—perhaps heirloom fruits and vegetables

- *Ripe-from-the-farm flavor*—especially when you pick it yourself
- *Samples to taste*
- *Market entertainment*—culinary demonstrations and local crafts
- *Growers' secrets*—on growing and selecting the best produce. Just ask; vendors will likely share a cooking tip or two, as well.

Find a farmer's market near you.

- *Read* your local newspaper, or call your county Cooperative Extension agent.
- *Call* the U.S. Department of Agriculture Farmers Market Hotline (800-384-8704) or visit www.ams.usda.gov/farmersmarkets.

June 17   Rate Your Plate

Wonder how your food choices rate? You could keep a food diary, then tally food-group servings, nutrients, and calories. That works, but there's an easier way—online.

The Interactive Healthy Eating Index (IHEI) from the U.S. Department of Agriculture does the calculating for you. Just enter what you ate for a day on its Web site. The nutrition calculator figures how your day's food choices match food-group recommendations, nutrient advice, or both for your age and gender. That includes calories, vitamins, minerals, and other nutrients and food substances, including those you may need to control: fat, saturated fat, cholesterol, and sodium.

Use the IHEI to quickly check your day's food choices or to follow the progress of your "eat smart" plan.

- *Click here:* www.usda.gov/cnpp for the IHEI.
- *Measure.* That's the key to any accurate nutrition feedback from computer analysis or written records. Get out the measuring cups and spoons if you need to.
- *Remember to include condiments and drinks.* They can supply hidden calories.

June 18 🏃 Fit for Hot Weather

Summer weather is no excuse to "chill out" indefinitely in your air-conditioned family room. The guideline still applies: Get 60 minutes of moderate activity every day if you can.

In the summer heat, try air-conditioned action, such as indoor mall walking or inside home improvement projects. Enjoy summertime sports such as swimming, bicycling, tennis, canoeing, or in-line skating.

Active outdoor leisure can include early-morning or late-afternoon walks, nature hikes, playing with your kids in the sprinkler. And remember outdoor chores, like gardening and car, bike, or dog washing.

For safety's sake in hot, steamy weather:

- *Dress for it.* Wear a hat to shade your head and light-colored, light-weight, loose-fitting clothes.
- *Stay hydrated.* Drink plenty of fluids. Even when you swim, you sweat.
- *Go easy. Wait until later in the day* if the heat, humidity, and air quality are potentially dangerous.
- *Wear sunscreen.*

June 19 ⚕ Hey, Guy!

Do you like pizza, spaghetti with tomato sauce, burritos laden with salsa, lots of catsup, or old-fashioned tomato soup? Then enjoy 'em! Tomatoes are an abundant source of lycopene, a powerful antioxidant that may help reduce prostate cancer risk. Aside from skin cancer, prostate cancer is the most commonly diagnosed cancer in men in the United States, and the second leading cause of men's cancer death.

Two other antioxidants—selenium in fish, seafood, poultry, whole grains, and soybeans; and vitamin E in nuts—also *may* reduce prostate cancer risk. Some studies suggest protective substances in soybeans. Try soy beverages, soy nuts, soy flour, tofu, tempeh; soy's not just for women!

The general cancer prevention guidelines: smart eating (variety of plant-based foods including fruits and vegetables, low-fat eating), healthy weight, active living, not smoking.

Men: Pay attention to prostate health, starting this weekend.

- *Enjoy more tomatoes and soy foods.*
- *Eat lean:* lean meats, plenty of whole-grain foods, fruits, and veggies, easy on fat.
- *Schedule a prostate cancer screening*—every year if you're 50 or older, sooner if you're African American or have a family history of prostate cancer.

June 20   Talk Turkey

Time-starved? If you need to prepare dinner in fast-food time, shop turkey: turkey breast tenderloin or steak, ground turkey, turkey franks, or turkey ham.

Turkey's a great choice for health reasons, too. It's very lean, with most of its *fat (mostly unsaturated)* in the skin. Consider: 3½ ounces of cooked white, skinless turkey has just 160 calories and 3 fat grams. Darker meat has more fat, but less than many red meat cuts. And turkey supplies plenty of *protein,* some *B vitamins* and *selenium,* and good amounts of *iron* and *magnesium.*

Use ground turkey in burgers, "meatloaf," lasagna, pasta sauce, tacos; turkey ham or sausage in omelets, quiche, pizza, sandwiches, salads.

During Turkey Lovers' Month, put turkey on your table.

Turkey Kebabs

¼ cup vegetable oil	2 medium zucchini, in chunks
¼ cup fresh lime juice	2 medium red peppers, seeded, in chunks
1 teaspoon chili powder	chunks
½ teaspoon garlic powder	2 medium red onions, peeled, in chunks
½ teaspoon salt	chunks
1½ pounds fresh boneless turkey breast or thighs, in 1-inch cubes	

Combine oil, lime juice, chili powder, garlic powder, and salt. Toss vegetables and turkey cubes in oil mixture to coat. Marinate for 1 hour. Thread turkey and vegetables onto skewers. Grill over medium heat for 10 to 15 minutes or until turkey reaches an internal temperature of 180°F. Makes 6 servings.

Source: The National Turkey Federation/Ontario Turkey Producers' Marketing Board

June 21   Cook Savvy—Herb-y Ways to Flavor

Shake the salt habit! Excite your taste buds with herbs instead. With little effort, you get plenty of sodium-free flavor.

Herb tips: Use 1 tablespoon of fresh herbs for 1 teaspoon dried. Cut fresh herbs finely to maximize their aroma and flavor.

Boost flavor with herbs today.

- *Flavor your water.* Add mint, lemongrass, or scented geranium leaves.
- *Perk up olive oil.* Simmer oil gently with rosemary, garlic, or chilies for 15 minutes. Refrigerate leftover oil; use within 10 days.
- *Rub on flavor.* Press an herb rub on meat, poultry, or fish before cooking. Try this combo: chopped parsley, garlic, pepper, salt, and mustard.
- *Toss with greens.* Add chopped fresh herbs to a salad.
- *Add herbs near the end of cooking.* Then their flavors won't cook out.
- *Season rice, pasta, eggs, mashed potatoes, veggies—even pizza.* Hold back on salt; use herbs instead.
- *Mix into dough or batter.* Try chives, garlic, rosemary, or other herbs.
- *Get under the skin.* Stuff fresh herbs—sage, tarragon, savory— between poultry skin and poultry meat, and inside the cavity, then roast.
- *"Sweeten" fruit.* Add mint, lavender, or rosemary to fruit salads, cobblers, and smoothies.

June 22   Food Bug Got You?

Had an upset stomach, diarrhea, or fever recently? Maybe it's from something you ate. Your summer picnic basket or backyard buffet is the perfect breeding ground for food-borne bacteria. An estimated

76 million Americans get sick from food each year, and about 5,000 die from it.

Should you call your doctor if you think food made you sick? Rest and plenty of fluids are usually the best treatment, but get a doctor's care when . . .

- Diarrhea is bloody.
- Vomiting or diarrhea is excessive.
- Three symptoms appear: stiff neck, severe headache, fever.
- A fatal illness is suspected from *Clostridium botulinum* or *Vibrio vulnificus.*
- The victim is a young child, an elderly adult, or someone with cancer, HIV/AIDS, or at high-risk for another reason.
- Symptoms persist.

To prevent picnic-time food-borne illness:

- *Wash your hands often.* Use a hand sanitizer at a picnic.
- *Keep raw meats (in well-sealed containers) and ready-to-eat foods separate,* perhaps in different picnic coolers.
- *Cook to proper inside temperature.* Pack a meat thermometer for safe grilling. (See January 27 for safe temperatures.)
- *Keep your cooler well chilled.* Keep the lid closed.
- *Keep perishable food chilled.* It shouldn't sit out of the cooler for longer than one hour.

June 23   Confused about Carbs?

Despite the high-protein craze and recent carbohydrate bashing, the consensus of nutrition science remains that carbohydrates should be your body's main energy source. The Institute of Medicine advises that children and adults consume 45 to 65 percent of their calories (energy) from carbohydrates. For a 2,000-calorie day, that's 225 to 325 carbohydrate grams daily.

Are carbohydrates fattening? Not inherently. What's fattening are excess calories from *any* source—carbohydrates, fat, protein—and alcohol!

Are the carbohydrates in pasta, vegetables, fruit, and candy different? In food, yes. As energy, no. Grain products and vegetables supply mostly complex carbs; fruit and candy provide mostly different types of sugars. Whole-grain foods, vegetables, and some fruits have fiber, too. Except for fiber, all carbohydrates are digested to simple sugars before they're absorbed and used for energy.

Top-line advice: Pick your carbs wisely so you also get their nutrient partners—vitamins and minerals—along with phytonutrients.

- *Make grain choices "whole" for more fiber.* Pick whole-wheat bread, oat cereal, or brown rice, for example.
- *Go for veggies and fruit.* Eat one more serving today of either one. Goal: five to nine servings a day.
- *Ease up on soda or candy.* Try one portion less than usual today.

June 24 🍴 Tripping Up

You've been going 24/7, but it's finally time for a summer vacation. Regional cuisine is a great way to get the "taste" of the locale, but watch out! With too much eating for entertainment, calories can add up.

To avoid tripping up as you enjoy food on your vacation:

- *Order your main meal for lunch.* Lunch portions tend to be smaller.
- *Pace yourself.* One hearty meal a day—even when the cuisine or restaurants lure you—is likely enough.
- *Search menus.* Look for regional vegetables, fruits, and perhaps seafood, not just the dessert specialties.
- *Give yourself leeway.* If you indulge on vacation, leave feelings of guilt behind. Just get back on track with smart eating when you get home.

June 25 🍎 Hot Tomato

The French called tomatoes "apples of love." American colonists believed they were poisonous. Today the average American eats 90 pounds of tomatoes a year!

And today we know a juicy tomato is loaded with positive nutrition: two antioxidant vitamins—*vitamin C* and *beta carotene* (which forms vitamin A)—and a natural plant substance called lycopene. *Lycopene,* which makes tomatoes red, may be the most powerful antioxidant in the carotenoid family.

That's why tomatoes are so good for you. These antioxidants may help protect you from many cancers. Wondering about canned tomatoes? Once heat-processed or cooked, tomatoes deliver even more lycopene!

Store fresh tomatoes at room temperature to keep their full flavor and best texture.

Easy No-Cook Tomato Sauce

1 pound (3 to 4 medium) fresh tomatoes, coarsely chopped	2 teaspoons balsamic vinegar
1 tablespoon olive oil	¾ teaspoon each salt and sugar
	½ teaspoon ground pepper

In a food processor or blender, combine and process all ingredients to make a rough-textured sauce. Adjust flavors to taste. Makes about 1½ cups sauce.

Variations to add to finished sauce:

- ¼ cup chopped fresh basil
- ¼ cup chopped olives and 1½ teaspoons finely grated orange peel
- ½ cup crumbled feta cheese and ¾ teaspoon finely chopped fresh or dried rosemary
- 3 tablespoons toasted pine nuts and 5 thin slices prosciutto, chopped

Source: California Tomato Commission

June 26 Go Exotic for Five a Day

Cherimoya, feijoa, pepino: Sound foreign? They're specialty fruits. This National Fresh Fruit and Vegetable Month is the time to enjoy them both for their flavor and their nutrient and phytonutrient benefits.

Enjoy exotic fruits over ice cream, frozen yogurt, or even cereal; in a fruit smoothie or salad; or by themselves for their unique flavor.

Try one or more of these specialty fruits today:

- *Cactus pear,* or prickly pear, is the sweet, mild fruit of cactus plants. Peel; remove the seeds.
- *Cherimoya* (chair-oh-MOY-ah), or custard apple, has a custard-like consistency and flavor. Cut in half, remove seeds, and scoop out the fruit.

- *Feijoa* (fay-YOH-ah or fay-JOH-ah) looks like a kiwifruit without fuzz.
- *Guava* (GWAH-vah), sweet and fragrant, ranges from white- to red-fleshed. Enjoy whole if you like.
- *Kiwano* (kee-WAH-noh), orange and spiked outside, is juicy and green inside, and tastes like cucumber, banana, and lime.
- *Loquat,* a small tart fruit, is eaten whole. Remove the pit.
- *Pepino* is fragrant, with a juicy sweet yellow flesh. Peel first.
- *Persimmon* looks like a tomato. It's sweet when ripe, but bitter and sour when it's not.
- *Starfruit,* or carambola, forms a star when sliced.

June 27   Exercise Your Heart

Your heart beats faster and faster as your exercise gets more and more strenuous. Why? It's pumping more oxygen, so your body can produce more and more energy. Like leg and arm muscles, your heart muscle needs regular workouts. But how fast is safe and healthy?

Your target heart rate—beats per minute (bpm)—during a workout is a range, not one number. A healthy goal depends on your age, health, and fitness level.

Here's how to calculate your target range—if you're healthy. First calculate your maximum heart rate: 220 minus your age. Your target heart rate is 50 to 75 percent of maximum heart rate.

If you have a health problem, check with your doctor.

During your next physical activity, check your bpm (pulse) several times. Here's how:

- *First, feel the beat.* Put your fingers lightly but firmly (not too much pressure) on your neck just under your jaw, or inside your wrist.
- *Then count for 10.* Count your heartbeats for 10 seconds. Multiply that number by 6 for your bpm.
- *Last compare it to your target.*

Another option: Wear an electronic sensing device that tracks your heart rate.

June 28 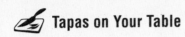 Tapas on Your Table

Looking for a relaxing eating adventure that can be as flavorful as it is nutritious? Try tapas!

Spanish tapas likely originated as street food. Served cold or hot, today these little plates of food are made with a limitless variety of high-quality ingredients—mostly without much effort, but with plenty of flavor and an array of nutrient-rich foods.

With tapas you can explore and savor many flavors easily.

For casual summer entertaining, have a tapas party at home.

- *Prepare tapas ahead—or ask each guest to bring one:* perhaps garlic broiled shrimp, herbed bread or focaccia, roasted almonds, marinated olives and mushrooms, proscuitto wrapped around salmon or asparagus, or potato tapas. (See February 4 and March 16.)
- *Serve tapas one at a time.* Offer wine, fruit juice, or bottled water to go with them.
- *Eat until you're satisfied,* not until you're overfull.
- *Have a good time, as the Spanish do,* as you slowly enjoy food and friends!

June 29   Get Real Simple

Energy drained? No time just for you? Too many choices? Maybe it's time to balance, to simplify. Some say, "Live simply so you can simply live." After all, balanced living is good not only for your head, but for your whole body.

Get "real simple" to put more balance—and more fitness—in your life.

- *Just say "no."* Let go, or at least cut back, on one thing you do. For example, bring a watermelon, not a homemade dessert, to a group picnic.
- *Delegate.* Divide family household duties: cooking, cleaning up, taking out garbage. Get more enthusiasm by letting others choose their tasks.
- *Find quicker ways to get things done.* Double batch for two meals at a time: chili for today, later chili-topped spuds. Buy partly

prepared foods to cut kitchen time. Let your slow cooker cook for you. Prepare meals on weekends; freeze until you need them.

- *Clean kitchen cabinets, drawers, and shelves.* Donate extras to a local shelter.
- *Deal once with papers, voice mail, clipped recipes and coupons, e-mail.* Off your desk, off your mind.
- *Decide what you don't need to do today—or maybe ever.* Try instead to accomplish one or two things well today.
- *Read April 15 and May 22 again!*

June 30   Cut Trans Fats

Shopping for groceries this week? Go easy on foods with trans fatty acids, found in many processed foods.

What makes them unhealthy? Processing these plant-based fats has made them saturated. Trans fatty acids may boost harmful LDL-blood cholesterol levels, perhaps more than other saturated fats do, while lowering protective HDL-cholesterol.

How much trans fat is okay? The National Academy of Sciences (NAS) advises that you keep trans fatty acids as low as you can. They have no known health benefits.

How low can you go? Opting out completely isn't practical since they're in so many types of foods and some are naturally found in food. With an all-out ban you'd probably find it too hard to get the other nutrients you need.

Cut back on trans fats by knowing where they hide.

- *Check ingredients on food labels for partially hydrogenated oils.* Hydrogenation turns unsaturated vegetable fats into trans fats. Some foods with trans fats: margarine, cookies, frosting, snack cakes, pastry, pie crust. More and more foods list trans fats on the Nutrition Facts.
- *Look for food products labeled "trans fat free."*
- *Eat more of foods with few, if any, trans fats:* fruit, vegetables, whole-grain foods, fish, lean meat and poultry, nuts, and olive, canola, and safflower oils.

July 1   🧬 Another Reason to Keep Trim

If you're trying to keep your weight in a healthy range, or looking for another motivation to do so, consider this: We've long known that obesity ups the risk for heart disease, diabetes, and high blood pressure, as well as cancer.

Now experts say that mounting evidence suggests a link to cancer is more than poor diet and inactivity. Obesity itself—the amount of body fat—may play a role. Perhaps extra hormones, produced by body fat, encourage cell growth, more rapid cell division, and with them, perhaps, cell mutations. Or maybe it's linked to body fat's ability to store cancer-causing substances before they're removed from the body.

Whatever the reason, obesity increases breast cancer risk among women and colon cancer risk among both genders, especially men. Other cancers are also associated with obesity.

Commit—or recommit—yourself to a healthy weight today. If you're not at your healthy weight, even taking off a few pounds can make a health difference. Two slimming tips to remember:

- *Slim down your food portions.*
- *Take a brisk walk today*—and nearly every day.

July 2   🍎 Can't Beet 'Em!

For their color splash and health benefits, beets—both the root and the greens—are hard to beat! Their color is a sure sign of antioxidant benefits.

Fresh or canned, beets are good for you: just 50 calories in a medium-size beet, almost no fat, and a good source of *folate, potassium, fiber,* and health-promoting *antioxidants.* Eat fresh beet greens, too—especially now that they're in season. Compared with the root, a half-cup serving of greens has double the *potassium,* and it's high in *beta carotene* (which forms vitamin A).

Tip: As you prepare beets, wear gloves and use a cutting board so your hands and countertop won't stain.

Put ruby-colored beets on your table today: sliced or grated fresh beets in stir-fries, beet greens or canned beets in salads.

Mustard-Roasted Vegetable Medley

1 large parsnip, peeled and juli-enned (cut in thin matchsticks)	1 tablespoon prepared mustard
1 large carrot, peeled and julienned	1½ teaspoons maple syrup
1 large beet, peeled and julienned	1 teaspoon oil
	Salt and pepper to taste

Heat oven to 450°F. Coat a small oven-proof pan with nonstick cooking spray. Toss all ingredients until well combined. Bake, stirring occasionally, about 20 minutes or until vegetables are tender. Makes 2 servings.

Source: Vegetarian Resource Group

July 3 ✍ Sundae, Sweet Sundae

I scream, we scream—do *you* scream for ice cream? Ninety percent of United States households buy ice cream, and we average about five gallons per person yearly.

But which ice cream? Premium has richer flavor, yet more fat and calories. Choose reduced-fat, low-fat, light, or fat-free if you're cutting back on fat; lactose-free, if you're lactose intolerant; or calcium-rich, for more calcium.

Smart alternatives are frozen yogurt (whole, low-fat, or fat-free), with or without live, active cultures, and fruit sorbet or soy frozen dessert if you're a strict vegetarian.

Celebrate July, Ice Cream Month, with a great sundae.

- *Enjoy a sensible-size sundae.* Find the calories in a serving (usually ½ cup) on a frozen dessert label. Is your portion larger than a serving? Surprised?
- *Make it fruit-full.* Spoon ice cream between layers of mango, papaya, blueberries, kiwi, or figs.
- *Go nuts.* A small handful of pistachios, pine nuts, hazelnuts, or almonds sprinkled on top will bump up the phytonutrient benefits.

July 4   Grilling? Flavor Your Fourth

Grilling again? Because grilling is a low-fat way to cook, it's healthy—and can make healthful food even tastier.

Try these hints to add flavor, yet no fat or salt:

- *Marinate veggies as well as meat, poultry, and fish.* Marinate with oil-and-vinegar dressing in a zip-top plastic bag for quick cleanup.
- *Time your basting.* Brush on light, oil-based sauces earlier in grilling. For less charring, baste sauces containing sugars (fruit purée, honey, preserves) toward the end of the cooking.
- *Grill veggies.* Just brush on a little olive oil and herbs first.
- *Smoke it.* Brush on a little liquid smoke. It adds more outdoor taste, and it's safe to eat.
- *Season your coals.* Toward the ending of grilling, sprinkle flavorful fresh herbs, citrus or apple peels, even whole, unpeeled garlic cloves on your coals. Enjoy the delicate flavor this gives.
- *For safety's sake:* Turn back to May 25 for more tips on grilling safely.

July 5   Take a Walking or a Biking Tour

Enjoy walking or biking as a regular routine? Then sign up for a walking, hiking, or biking tour—around town, in a domestic vacation destination, or even in a foreign country.

If your regular route seems boring or tedious, taking your feet or bike on tour can divert your mind and introduce new surroundings. Perhaps best of all, a walking or biking tour gives you freedom to explore nooks and crannies and see sights from a unique, close-up perspective. With a good workout, too, your independence gives you a great chance to find local foods to recharge your personal battery.

Take time today to find a local or distant place to stretch and pump your legs.

- *Search the Internet for walking vacation tours*—a specialty for some travel companies.
- *Find a tour that matches your level of physical fitness.*

July 6   Follow the Rainbow

Did you reach for at least one red or pink fruit or vegetable today? How about dark green, deep yellow, or orange? Purple or blue? For good health, the more color on your plate, the better.

Those colors come from thousands of phytonutrients, which independently or together promote health.

- *Green:* Lutein in broccoli, collards, green peas, and spinach may help reduce the chances of macular degeneration and cataracts. Indoles in some green veggies may help reduce prostate and breast cancer risk.
- *Deep yellow/orange:* Beta carotene in carrots, pumpkin, sweet potatoes, peaches, and mangoes may help slow aging, reduce the chances of cancer and heart disease, and give your immune system a boost.
- *Purple/blue:* Anthocyanins in blackberries, blueberries, eggplant, plums, and purple grapes may help reduce cancer risk and perhaps help prevent urinary tract infections.
- *Red:* In tomatoes, red cabbage, sweet cherries, strawberries, pink grapefruit, and watermelon, lycopene helps protect against prostate cancer. Many of these foods have anthocyanins, too.
- *White:* Allyl sulfides in garlic, leeks, and onions may help control cholesterol and blood pressure and help your body fight infection.

Reach for the "color-coded" benefits of fruits and vegetables today.

- *Think five-a-day twice today:* Eat at least five fruit and vegetable servings, and try to put five colors in your meals and snacks, too.
- *Eat the colorful peels,* too, if they're edible.

July 7   Pack a Healthful Picnic

What's for tonight's dinner? Why not pack a picnic cooler before work, so it's ready to go when you are.

- *Keep clean.* Bring hand wipes or sanitizer, a clean tablecloth, and separate utensils for preparing and for eating.

- *Keep cold food cold.* If perishable (meat, poultry, fish, eggs, mayonnaise), keep your food in a chilled cooler. Don't store your cooler in a hot car.
- *Keep bug free.* Put food in well-sealed containers.

This summer, remember to make your picnic simple, safe, and savory.

- *Go vegetarian:* a hearty salad (beans, cooked rice or pasta, and chopped vegetables, tossed with an herb vinaigrette), peach or mango, and breadsticks.
- *Keep it easy:* several cheeses, hearty whole-grain bread, grapes and berries, zucchini sticks, and calamata olives.
- *Toss it there:* canned tuna, canned pineapple chunks or mandarin oranges, chopped bell pepper, banana slices, toasted almonds, chives, and low-fat mayonnaise (a small jar, unopened) served on fresh greens. (*Tip:* Remember the can opener.)
- *Remember drinks:* juice or water, perhaps frozen ahead to stay cold as they melt.

July 8   🍒 Just a Bowl of Cherries

Life may be "just a bowl of cherries" as the old song says. On the flip side: Cherries may help promote life!

It's cherry season; choose plump, sweet Rainiers or deep-red Bings. Cherries contain not only *fiber* and some *vitamin C.* As part of healthful eating and living, other substances in cherries—*anthocyanins, quercetin,* among others—may offer sweet benefits, too, promoting heart health, reducing cancer risk, and perhaps reducing arthritis symptoms or pain. And their natural *melatonin* may even help put you to sleep. What a cheery, cherry thought!

Today, or any time of year, put cherries in your life.

- *Refresh with a cherry-berry smoothie:* Blend equal amounts of frozen or canned cherries, frozen strawberries, and cran-cherry juice drink.
- *Add fresh or dried cherries to slaw, precut greens, or spinach salad.*

Cherry and Hazelnut Salad

1 pound fresh sweet cherries, pitted* and sliced
6 cups mixed lettuces
¾ cup crumbled Gorgonzola cheese
½ cup chopped toasted hazelnuts
⅓ cup vinaigrette salad dressing, homemade or purchased

In a large bowl, combine cherries, lettuces, cheese, and hazelnuts. Just before serving, drizzle salad with vinaigrette and toss lightly. Makes 6 servings.

Source: Washington State Fruit Commission/Northwest Cherries

*A cherry pitter makes it easy!

July 9 Write Your Own Best-seller

Looking for the latest, greatest diet book? Rather than scan bookstore shelves for a trendy weight-loss plan with solutions from others, "author" a plan devised uniquely for you. As your personal best-seller, successful weight management needs to match your own health needs—and your own food, lifestyle, and active living preferences.

Most weight problems come from excess: excess calories, excess portions, excess inactivity. But we each take our own road to get there—we each need our own solutions, too.

For the right-for-you action plan:

- *First consider what you've tried in the past:* what worked, what didn't work over several months, and why.
- *Judge it for yourself:* What could I change to stick with it? What steps did I take then to control my portions, trim calories, eat a variety of healthful food? What can I do differently now? What physical activities did I do and do I like to do? What am I doing right now—and what not?
- *Write your best-selling strategies,* a weight-loss approach with you in mind. Follow general guidelines of healthful eating (see January 15 and 16) and active living. And contact a registered dietitian (RD) if you need a "writing" coach. (See March 1.)

July 10 Beer Here!

Iced drinks taste great on a hot summer day. Wonder if a cold beer could be good for you, too?

Drinking beer *in moderation* may offer healthful side effects, perhaps as much as wine. Beer *may* provide some protection against diabetes, high blood pressure, heart attack, and stroke—more likely from its ethanol than from its modest amounts of B vitamins. Moderation is key to any health benefits: no more than one drink daily for women, two for men. (A drink is 12 ounces beer, 5 ounces wine, or 1½ ounces distilled spirits.)

Downing a six-pack negates any benefits. Binge drinking increases the chances of obesity, liver failure, stroke, and some cancers. For the record, a 12-ounce regular beer has 150 calories; a six-pack (12 ounces each), 900!

If you enjoy beer in moderation, consider this during July, American Beer Month:

- *Pair beer with food.* Choose the beer that pairs well for flavor: *full-bodied ale* with hearty dishes and meat, *hoppier beer* with spicy foods, and light beer with salads, seafood, and light sandwiches.
- *Go beyond beer tradition. Choose from*
    "Low-carb" beer—fewer calories, less carbohydrates, and perhaps slightly less alcohol
    Low-alcohol or reduced-alcohol beer
    Alcohol-free malt beverage
    Flavored malt beverage—with juice, fruit, or fruit concentrate added. Still, go easy.

July 11   Park Here

Day walks, night walks, bird watching, horseback riding, canoeing, white-water rafting, and more—local, state, and national parks have plenty going on. Take advantage of events geared to keep you moving.

Enjoy all that parks have to offer during Recreation and Parks Month and at every season of the year.

- *Take your picnic on a hike.* Why spend the afternoon sitting at the picnic grounds near the parking lot?

- *Check the park calendar.* Sign up for a scheduled nature walk with the conservationist or an archeological walk in a historical park.
- *Sign up as a park volunteer.* Tasks you do are often physically active.
- *Walk trails, beaches, and riverbanks for cleanup*—great way to teach environmental responsibility to kids.

July 12 Staying Fit—It's an Attitude

Attitude is everything! You probably heard that from your parents and teachers when you were growing up. An attitude of personal control over body weight seems to increase the chance of success. That makes sense. To stay motivated, most people need to feel they're in control and that what they do makes a difference. Fact is, even people genetically programmed to carry more weight can have healthy, fit bodies.

To keep a "fit" attitude:

- *Learn to love your body, heavy or thin.* You'll be more willing to care for it.
- *Shift your focus away from food and the scale.* Tune in to interests that don't include food.
- *Enjoy positive self-talk.* Think about all you *can* do. Apply that same attitude to healthful eating and staying physically active.

July 13 Organic—or Not?

You've probably noticed that stores and produce markets have more varieties of organic food than ever, with plenty of good quality. Are their benefits worth any extra cost? That's your call.

As shopping alternatives, scientific evidence doesn't show that organic foods are safer, healthier, or more nutritious. The flavor? Some consumers perceive a flavor difference, which likely comes from the type of food rather than from the way it was grown.

What does organic labeling, regulated by the U.S. Department of Agriculture, mean?

- *100 percent organic*—made only with organic ingredients
- *Organic*—made with at least 95 percent organic ingredients
- *Made with organic ingredients*—must contain at least 70 percent organic ingredients

To clarify: Organic foods aren't necessary grown without pesticides or fertilizers, but instead with those types found naturally in the environment, with substances on an approved list, or with insects that are natural predators.

If you prefer organically produced foods:

- *Try a new varietal.* Local organic farmers may produce interesting and flavorful heirloom vegetables and fruits.
- *Read organic labeling.* Be sure you get what you are looking for.

July 14 🩺 X-File—Stay Out!

If X marks the spot, just what is syndrome X? And do you need to be concerned? The Centers for Disease Control and Prevention estimates that 22 percent of adults, especially older adults, have it.

Syndrome X, or insulin resistance, is really four health conditions—diabetes, high blood pressure, unhealthy blood lipid levels (high triglycerides, low HDL- [good] cholesterol), and obesity—that all come together. When that happens, heart disease, heart attack, and stroke risks are many times higher.

With syndrome X, the body doesn't react normally to insulin, so more is produced. That contributes to high blood pressure, insulin buildup, glucose intolerance, and unhealthy lipid levels. Inactivity, overeating, and overweight aggravate the insulin problem.

If you think you're at risk:

- *Get your numbers checked:* blood sugar level, lipid level, blood pressure. (See July 21 for normal ranges.) Work out a plan with your doctor to bring them within normal range.
- *Make a realistic plan to trim a few pounds*—if you're overweight.
- *Move more.* Try to fit 60 minutes—even in small intervals—of moderate activity into your day.
- *Eat plenty of high-fiber foods:* whole grains, vegetables, fruit.

July 15 🍎 Berry, Berry Good for You

July marks the height of fresh blueberry season. So tuck a carton of blueberries in your shopping cart.

Why so "berry" good? *Anthocyanins,* which give their deep-blue hue, add more than color. Along with *vitamin C,* anthocyanins and *other phenolics* are among the many health-promoting antioxidants in these sweet berries. Antioxidants may protect your body cells from damage that can lead to heart disease, cancer, and other health problems. And anthocyanins may protect against urinary tract infections. Blueberries also contain *fiber* and *ellagic acid,* thought to be cholesterol-lowering and cancer protective.

Try blueberries (fresh, frozen, or canned) in smoothies, seafood or chicken salads, as garnishes on poultry, fish, and pork—or in a "berry" easy dessert.

Dessert Waffles with Spiced Blueberry Sauce

2 cups fresh blueberries, divided
3 tablespoons sugar
4 teaspoons cornstarch
1 teaspoon ground cinnamon
¼ to ½ teaspoon ground black
   pepper

⅓ cup water
4 fresh or frozen (4½-inch) waffles
4 scoops vanilla frozen yogurt or
   ice cream

In a small saucepan, combine half of the blueberries with the sugar, cornstarch, cinnamon, black pepper, and water. Bring to a boil over medium heat; boil for 1 minute. Remove from heat and stir in remaining blueberries; cool. Toast waffles; place on dessert plates. Scoop frozen yogurt onto waffles; top with blueberry sauce. Makes 4 servings.
Source: U.S. Highbush Council

July 16 🌾 Right-Size for Fitness

Despite the commitment and the discipline to eat smart and stay active, keeping trim is easier for some, harder for others. Today health experts understand that there is no perfect size, shape, or weight. What's really important is being healthy with the body that's yours.

Make a plan to right-size yourself for fitness.

- *Set a date for a physical checkup.*
- *Monitor your health numbers:* cholesterol, trigylcerides, blood pressure, blood sugar level. Keep them within a healthy range.
- *Find a way—your way—to be physically active each day.*
- *Learn to control your portions.* If you tend to overeat, perhaps keep food out of sight so it's out of mind.
- *Eat for variety:* perhaps more fruits, vegetables, and whole-grain foods; enough dairy and protein-rich foods; fewer high-calorie, high-fat foods.
- *Make your weight goal realistic and healthy—for you!*

July 17   Summertime, and the Eatin' Is Easy

Food-filled festivals—such delicious, but potentially high-calorie (high-fat, high-sugar) fun. Funnel cakes, French fries, and soda add up!

If outdoor food festivals become your regular summer fare:

- *Eat a light meal beforehand.* It will help control your appetite at the festival.
- *Bring your own street food:* whole fruit, trail mix, canned juice, bottled water.
- *Check out the options before you buy.* Look for healthful options: fruit in a cup, a grilled turkey drumstick, frozen yogurt.
- *Split an order of festival food.* If you share, you share the calories with someone else, too.
- *Gravitate toward festival activities that get you moving:* interactive fun, walking to see craft booths.

July 18   In the Mood

Feel down? In a funk? Even a short interval of physical activity might be the mood booster you need! Research shows that regular physical activity may help reduce stress and may lower the chances of—or speed the relief of—depression.

What's the exercise link to mental health? The reasons aren't clear. But it might be partly chemical: perhaps more endorphins released in the brain, or more phenylethylamine (a natural amphetamine) released with aerobic movement. Or maybe it's the feeling of accomplishment that comes with meeting a fitness goal or the distraction from stress-provoking events.

Let the mood-boosting benefits get you in the mood to move today!

- *Fit in at least 10 active minutes of walking today.* Then work up to 60 minutes—regularly!
- *Get going with a friend.* Camaraderie is mood-boosting, too.

July 19 🍎 Get a Little "Culture"

You're told to protect against disease-causing bacteria: wash your hands, refrigerate perishable food, cook food thoroughly, keep food clean. Then what are friendly bacteria?

Probiotics are health-promoting bacteria that grow naturally in your intestines, and help keep fungi and harmful bacteria there at bay. If antibiotics wipe them out, there's nothing to keep the bad guys in check. Potential problem? Perhaps diarrhea.

Friendly bacteria—*Lactobacillus* and *Bifiodobacterium*—live in some yogurts and fermented milks. Ingesting good bacteria may sustain or reintroduce good bacteria in your gut. That's why your doctor may suggest yogurt or milk with active cultures if you have a gastrointestinal (GI) upset. Good bacteria also may help with lactose intolerance, improve immunity, and perhaps reduce your risk of cancer or a high cholesterol level.

For a little "culture" in your meals:

- *Look for "contains live cultures" on the label.* Your best bet: some yogurts, kefir (a fermented milk), and some acidophilus milk. If it says *"made with* live cultures," processing may have destroyed the bacteria.
- *Be cautious of probiotic supplements.* Take them only with guidance from your health care professional.

- *Be sensible.* Probiotics won't cure an ongoing GI problem. Get medical attention.

July 20   🛒 Cooking from "Speed-Scratch"

Want homemade flavor in fast-food time? "Speed-scratch" cooking may be your answer. Just toss together one or two fresh foods with a couple of packaged products that may be already cut up, cooked, or mixed with other flavorful, nutritious ingredients.

Spawned by consumer research, all kinds of high-flavor, nutrient-rich speed-scratch products have been launched. In the 1980s consumers looked for everyday recipes with 10 to 20 ingredients, to prepare in 45 minutes or less. Today, it's often three to five ingredients, prepared in 15 minutes or less.

Keep nutrient-rich "speed scratch" ingredients on hand! Check the Nutrient Facts to know the calories and nutrients in a serving.

- *Pocket salad:* mixed greens (bag), roasted red peppers (jar), marinated artichoke hearts (can), stuffed in a pita pocket.
  Grilled chicken with corn salsa: grilled chicken breast, topped with a combination of green or red salsa (jar), Mexican-style corn with chilies (can), and fresh cilantro
- *Pork stir-fry:* precut pork cubes (refrigerated or frozen) cooked and stirred with stir-fry veggies (frozen) and teriyaki sauce (bottle), served over rice

July 21   ⚕ Know Your Numbers?

Your age, gender, or family history—you can't control those risks for health problems. But your health numbers are a different story. Talk to your doctor about risk factors you may have and about what health-screening tests and exams you need and when. Then eat smart, stay active, and follow sound medical advice to manage your health before your numbers become risk factors for ongoing health problems.

	Normal or Optimal	Your Numbers Date _____	Your Numbers Date _____	Your Numbers Date _____
Total blood cholesterol	below 200 mg/dL			
HDL blood cholesterol	more than 60 mg/dL			
LDL blood cholesterol	below 100 mg/dL			
Triglycerides	below 150 mg/dL			
Blood pressure*	below <120/<80 mm Hg			
Fasting blood sugar	between 70 and 110 mg/dL			
Body mass index	between 18.5 and 24.9			

*Prehypertension: a range of 120/80 to 139/89

Take care of you:

- *Call for an appointment today* if you aren't up-to-date with your routine checkups.
- *Numbers not optimal?* If you've slipped off your personal care plan, take stock of the challenges and make a new plan that does work for you.

July 22 ✍ Your Nose Knows

Close your eyes and imagine the aromas: bread baking in the oven, fresh herbs crushed in your fingers, a ripe summer melon.

Smell is a remarkable ability. Not only do aromas evoke memories of times and places, smell also contributes to about 80 percent of food's flavor. The rest comes from a food's taste and texture.

Savor the aromas of summer at the table.

- *Decorate with bouquets of fresh herbs:* lemon mint, scented geranium, lavender, lemon verbena, or bergamot. You can also use them for cooking.
- *Make an aromatic sun tea* with citrus peel, cinnamon, mint, or other herbs.
- *Warm bakery-fresh bread* to go with summer soup or salad, to bring out its aroma.

July 23   Cooking Savvy—Recipe Makeovers

Want to enjoy your favorite high-calorie dishes? You can! With a quick makeover they can deliver even more health-promoting benefits than before.

To transform your favorite recipes for less fat and calories and more nutrition:

- *Make portions smaller.* A half portion of macaroni and cheese, fettucini alfredo, or chilies relleno has half the fat and calories.
- *Add health-promoting ingredients.* Add sweet potatoes to stew, broccoli to pizza, sun-dried tomatoes to mac and cheese, or sweet peppers to potato salad.
- *Substitute.* Sauté in olive oil rather than butter or margarine. Use evaporated fat-free milk in place of cream, and plain yogurt instead of sour cream.
- *Switch the food prep method.* Keep edible peels on vegetables and fruits. Oven-bake breaded chicken or shoestring potatoes, rather than fry them.

July 24   No Mistake about It

Committed to physical activity? Great, but watch out for common *mistakes* that even fit-minded people make.

- *No warmup, little pre- and post-stretching, no cool-down.* Warming up, then stretching prepares your heart and muscles for the core of your workout. Cool-down brings your heart rate down gradually and keeps your muscles from feeling stiff.
- *Intensity: too much or too little.* Forget "no pain, no gain." Longer, moderate exercise usually gives more fitness and healthy weight benefits; soreness often leads to quitting.
- *Drinking too little.* Drink enough to stay hydrated and move at your physical best. The best fluid replacer: plenty of water!
- *Equipment misuse.* Jerking or lifting too much weight can cause injury and pain. Slow, controlled movement and progressive strength training are safer and more effective.

Simple reminders for today's workout:

- *Drink enough.*
- *Warm up, then stretch for 10 minutes; cool down and stretch for 10 minutes.*
- *Try to fit in 60 minutes of moderate activity today*—even if you need to do it in smaller intervals.
- *Use equipment properly.* Ask for advice if you need to.

July 25 And the Facts Are . . .

Imagine you're comparing two supplements. Which one will you buy?

Start with the label. Supplement Facts and ingredient declarations on supplement containers look much like what's on food labels.

You will find percent Daily Values (DVs) if the nutrient is present or if a claim is made about it. If an ingredient has no DV (perhaps omega-3 fatty acids or an herbal), just the quantity in a serving (dose) is listed.

You won't find standardized dosages or potency. You likely can't discern active ingredients.

A supplement container may display three types of claims. Science backs up U.S. Food and Drug Administration (FDA)-approved nutrient and health claims. But structure/function claims, such as "echinacea boosts the immune system," aren't FDA approved; research behind these claims is limited, without scientific agreement.

Another guide—a certifying mark, such as USP—may verify the contents. These marks aren't FDA regulated, and criteria differ from mark to mark. They don't mean a supplement is "safe and effective."

The supplement savvy:

- *Remember food first!* A supplement is simply a supplement.
- *Stay sensible.* 100% DV for nutrients is enough.
- *Talk to your doctor.* Ask whether and how much is safe for you.
- *Contact supplement manufacturers* for documentation of label information and claims.

July 26   🍎 So Corn-y

Ready to smile from ear to ear? Enjoy summer-fresh corn on the cob—the fresher, the sweeter! When corn gets picked, its natural sugar starts changing to starch.

Whether fresh, frozen, or canned, corn often gets overlooked for its health benefits. Besides being a great source of *complex carbs* and fiber, yellow corn has plenty of *zeaxanthin* and cancer-fighting *lutein*. These plant substances (phytonutrients) in the carotenoid family also may help promote heart health and normal vision and may protect you in the long run from macular degeneration.

Since it's peak corn season, enjoy some fresh-picked corn today.

- *Roast corn on the outdoor grill* for a gentle, smoky flavor. Soak it 30 minutes or so in the husk; grill husk-on.
- *Microwave it.* For moist corn in minutes, wrap each ear in wet paper towels or waxed paper first.
- *Cook a few extra ears.* Remove the kernels and enjoy in soup, salad, salsas, and stir-fries.

July 27   ⚕ Gas-tronomy

Like beans, but they don't like you? A high-fiber diet may cause intestinal gas. Drinking enough water may be enough of an antidote.

Need more relief? Check the pharmacy shelf. One of three types of products might help: (1) products with simethicone, which break large pockets of gas into smaller bubbles; (2) products with alpha-galactosidase, which convert gas-producing carbohydrates to more easily digested sugars, taken before a meal; and (3) products with charcoal, which help absorb intestinal gas, taken before or after a meal (not recommended for children, and may interfere with some medication).

Beans are loaded with health benefits (see February 20), so don't give them up. Just learn how to tame the reaction.

If you "gas up," try this:

- *After soaking dried beans, toss the water.* Some gas-producing carbohydrates dissolve into the soaking water. Cook in fresh water.
- *Cook dried, soaked beans thoroughly.* They'll digest easier.
- *Drain and rinse canned beans.* (It gets rid of some sodium, too.)

July 28   Passport to Health—Eating Caribbean Style

The term "barbecue" came from the Caribbean-Indian term *barbacoa*. Besides its delicious barbecue, Caribbean cooking features a nourishing array of tropical ingredients: a rainbow of fruits, rich in vitamin C, beta carotene, and other phytonutrients; the pear-shaped avocado with its monounsaturated fatty acids, vitamins, and phytonutrients; a bounty of warm-water seafood with less saturated fat than meat; the "combo" of rice and peas or beans, which together deliver complex carbs, protein, and fiber; and starchy tubers (yautia, yuca, yam, taro) with less familiar names.

Enjoy nourishing Caribbean flavors to complement today's hot-weather meal.

- *Go tropical* with guava, mango, papaya, pineapple, passion fruit.
- *Garnish with avocado or a lime squeeze* on salads, fish, and soups.
- *Jerk the flavor!* Rub peppery jerk seasoning on lean meat, seafood, or poultry before grilling. Buy jerk blend, or make your own.

Caribbean Jerk Rub

2 tablespoons dried minced onion	2 teaspoons ground allspice
1 tablespoon garlic powder	2 teaspoons black pepper
1 tablespoon sugar	1 teaspoon cayenne pepper
4 teaspoons crushed dry thyme leaves	½ teaspoon ground nutmeg
2 teaspoons salt	½ teaspoon ground cinnamon

In a jar with a tight-fitting lid, shake together all spices and other seasonings. Store tightly covered at room temperature. Makes about ½ cup.

Source: National Pork Board

July 29 🌾🧀 Nutrition Data—A Click Away

Looking for iron-rich foods, or perhaps low-sodium foods? Wonder how the nutrition in soyburgers compares with beef burgers?

Food labels offer easy access to "top-line" nutrient and calorie data for one serving of any food. But what if you need more than the label's Nutrition Facts? Just log on to the Internet. The U.S. Department of Agriculture maintains an online National Nutrient Database with more than 6,000 food items.

For easy access to this nutrient database:

- *Click onto www.nal.usda.gov/fnic/foodcomp/.* You can scroll through the alphabetical food list, organized by food groups, and get information on about 30 nutrients for every food that's listed.
- *Download the information for easy use* on your personal computer or handheld personal digital assistant (PDA) with a Palm operating system.

July 30 🌾🧀 Cooked or Raw—Which Is Better?

Are raw foods better for you? Despite recent interest in raw-food diets, combining cooked and raw foods is a smarter approach. Proper cooking retains most nutrient levels, and the heating process makes some phytonutrients more available for digestion and absorption. For example:

- *Cancer-fighting carotenoids* in cooked or canned carrots
- *Lycopene,* a phytonutrient that may protect against prostate cancer, from cooked or canned tomatoes
- *Phenolics,* also antioxidants, in cooked or canned sweet corn

For those who claim that cooking destroys important enzymes in raw food, note: Enzymes in raw foods may be essential to a vegetable or a fruit, but not to humans. Your body makes its own.

Another benefit of cooking: heat destroys harmful bacteria in raw foods that may cause food-borne illness. When you do eat raw fruits and vegetables, always clean them well.

Enjoy a combination of cooked and raw foods today.

- *Crisp garden-fresh greens,* tossed with roasted bell pepper
- *Tropical fruit compote,* topped with toasted hazelnuts
- *Oven-baked sweet potato,* topped with fresh mango-mint salsa

July 31   What's Cooking with Kids

Are your kids or grandkids already bored with summer activities and looking for something new to do? (See June 11.) Then bring playtime into the kitchen.

Children feel important when they help prepare food for themselves and their family. They often eat foods they wouldn't otherwise when they help prepare them. Kitchen time can nurture close family bonds and lifelong memories as you cook, create, and taste together.

Get a children's cookbook from the library or bookstore, or go online for easy and fun children's recipes.

Together find kid-friendly recipes that match your child's skills. For starters, try these simple ideas:

- *Fruit smoothies.* Shake juice, milk or frozen yogurt, and ice in a sealed container.
- *Homemade pretzels.* Shape thawed, whole-wheat freezer dough into alphabet letters. Bake them.
- *Toaster pizza.* Top pita bread with tomato sauce, chopped veggies, and grated cheese. Help kids safely bake it in the toaster oven.
- *Bananas crunch.* Roll peeled bananas in peanut butter or yogurt and crushed cereal, then freeze.

August 1   Get Exotic, Go for Eggplant

Have you considered the exotic, deep-purple eggplant for your five-a-day vegetable and fruit servings? Though used in many recipes as a meat substitute, eggplant has little protein. But it's fiber-rich (especially with its edible peel), fat- and cholesterol-free, and low in calories—a half cup of cooked eggplant has about 15 calories! Kept chilled and cooked fresh, eggplant makes a mild (not bitter) dish.

Try this meal-in-a-dish as eggplant season peaks:

Pork-Stuffed Eggplant

1 medium eggplant
½ pound lean ground pork
1 small green pepper, coarsely chopped
¼ cup chopped onion
1 clove garlic, minced

¼ cup water
⅛ teaspoon dried oregano
⅛ teaspoon pepper
1 medium tomato, coarsely chopped

Preheat oven to 350°F. Wash eggplant; cut in half lengthwise. Remove pulp, leaving the eggplant shell about ¼-inch thick. Cut pulp into ½-inch cubes. Set shells and pulp aside. In a large skillet cook ground pork, green pepper, onion, and garlic until pork is browned; drain excess drippings. Add eggplant pulp, water, oregano, and pepper; cover and cook over low heat for 10 minutes, stirring occasionally. Remove from heat; stir in tomato. Spoon mixture into eggplant shells. Place in a 12-by-8-by-2-inch baking dish. Bake for 20 to 25 minutes or until heated through. Makes 2 servings.

Source: National Pork Board

August 2 Fridge Safety

How cold should your refrigerator be to keep food fresh and safe? Using the dial reading inside isn't enough to know if your fridge is cold enough. And you can't rely on how cold food feels. Besides, food may be spoiled long before it looks, smells, or tastes bad.

To avoid food-borne illness and keep harmful bacteria at bay, keep your refrigerator between 33° and 40°F. Above that, bacteria multiply fast. Like handwashing, thorough cooking, and kitchen cleanliness, a properly chilled refrigerator is a food safety essential.

Give your fridge a regular checkup:

- *Buy a refrigerator thermometer.* It's not costly. Put it in the center of the middle shelf. Set the temp below 40°F; check regularly.
- *Refrigerate food promptly.* Do it the minute you get home from shopping. The same goes for leftovers.
- *Keep the door closed.* Before opening the refrigerator door, decide what you need.
- *Keep the fridge clean.* Wipe spills immediately. Clean regularly with hot, soapy water, and rinse.
- *"Spring clean" weekly.* Toss expired foods.

- *Date leftovers.* In general, toss after four days.
- *In doubt about food's safety?* Throw it out!

August 3   High Five for Fiber

Fiber—you know you need it. In fact, health experts advise 21 to 38 fiber grams daily, depending on your age and gender. Can you give five reasons?

1. It keeps you "regular."
2. High-fiber foods fill you up, so you don't eat as much (good for weight watching).
3. Soluble fiber helps take cholesterol away (good for heart health).
4. Insoluble fiber may help protect against colorectal cancer.
5. Soluble fiber may help control blood sugar levels after a meal (good for those with diabetes).

Boost fiber today.

- *Buy high-fiber cereal.* One ounce may provide 10 fiber grams or more. To add 4 grams more, top with a half cup of raspberries.
- *Switch breads*—whole-grain versions of bread, bagels, rice, pita, tortillas. Whole-grain bread delivers 2 fiber grams per slice, compared with a half gram in a white bread slice.
- *Eat beans.* Try kidney, black, garbanzos, among others for at least 5 fiber grams per half cup. Try bean salsa, hummus made with garbanzos, or edamame (soybeans shelled or in the pod).
- *Eat "five a day"*—five to nine vegetable and fruit servings daily. Their fiber adds up.
- *Follow the $^2/_3$–$^1/_3$ guideline.* Fill your plate at least two-thirds full of fiber-rich veggies, fruits, and whole grains, and the rest with meat, poultry, or fish or other meat alternative.
- *Read February 6 again.*

August 4   Let's Dance

If the rhythm moves you, dance! You don't need to know fancy steps or have a partner. Even with two left feet you get the health-promoting benefits and the fun.

Especially if you get your heart pumping, dancing is great for heart and overall health. Sixty minutes of continuous dancing may burn 200 calories or more.

Dance your way to fitness sometime this week.

- *Go line dancing.* No partner needed, just move with the group.
- *Sign up for ethnic, ballroom, or swing dancing.* Find an adult ed class nearby.
- *Dance to your own music.* Just put on you favorite music (R&B, hip hop, jazz, whatever); move to the beat. To motivate yourself, indulge in a new CD.
- *Enjoy a dance class for singles.* Try aerobic, tap, modern dance— at the gym, YMCA, or other community center.
- *Find a "chair dancing" class*—a yoga-type workout using a chair for balance.
- *Skip the movies this weekend; go dancing instead!*

August 5   Food, Flavor, Fusion!

Feel artistic? Enjoy blending paints, musical notes, or words to express something new? Turn your creative genius toward the kitchen. Blend foods and flavors for more variety, new taste sensations, perhaps more nutrition.

"Fusion cuisine"— blending ingredients or cooking techniques of different cultures—is a culinary phenomenon. Though trendy, it's not new. Over time, every cuisine has been influenced by others to ultimately create its own ethnic distinction. Consider: Tomatoes that originated in the Americas transformed southern Italian cuisine over the past 500 years.

Create fusion dishes and give vegetables, fruits, and grain products a flavor boost.

- *Thai-Italian:* pizza crust coated with hoisin sauce, topped with sprouts, green onions, shredded carrots, cilantro, ginger, peanuts, and mild white cheese
- *Italian-Asian:* cooked pasta tossed with grilled chicken and Asian peanut sauce

- *French-Caribbean:* chocolate mousse topped with tropical fruit salsa
- *Italian-Southwest:* chili con carne, flavored with basil, topped with Parmesan cheese
- *Asian-American:* mashed sweet potatoes flavored with wasabi, or pumpkin soup flavored with curry powder
- *Mexican-Chinese:* Chinese stir-fry, wrapped in a warm flour tortilla

August 6   You're Kid-ing!

Got kids? If so, did you know that kids influence up to 80 percent of family food spending?

Still, as a family shopper, you control what foods go into the family kitchen. For children, you decide the three Ws: *What* foods to offer, *When*, and *Where*. As kids learn to be good eaters, they decide the other *W* and the *H*: *Which* offered foods to eat, *How much*. (Why "How much?" Kids need to learn to listen to their body cues, in order to know when they're really hungry and when they're full.)

As you shop for family foods:

- *Create the shopping list together.*
- *Stock food-group* snacks they like: perhaps fruit; crunchy veggies; pretzels; milk in kid-friendly containers; string cheese; single-serve fruit, yogurt drinks, or pudding snacks.
- *Shop supermarket aisles together.* Encourage children to pick fruits and vegetables they'd enjoy. Talk about foods' colors, shapes, and textures as you do.
- *Read food labels together.* That gives practice with reading skills, too.

August 7   Think Summer; Think Melon

Imagine: a blistering hot day with a slice of sweet, juicy watermelon—or an icy, thick smoothie made with fragrant cantaloupe or honeydew melon!

Melons are treasure troves—with more health-promoting benefits than simply water in the melon. Known for their *beta carotene* and *vitamin C,* melons have *vitamin B$_6$, potassium, magnesium,* and *thiamin,* as well as *fiber.* Watermelon also has plenty of cancer-fighting *lycopene.*

For fresh quality and best flavor, pick a watermelon heavy for its size, with a dry, brown stem. Thump it; the low-pitched sound suggests full, juicy flavor. For the sweetest flavor, pick cantaloupe with a fragrant perfume, netting on the rind, and a few tiny cracks near the stem. Try muskmelon, casaba, Crenshaw (half casaba, half Persian), or an exotic kiwano (horned melon), too.

Make your day "summer perfect" with melon.

Watermelon Fire and Ice Salsa

3 cups chopped watermelon
½ cup chopped green peppers
2 tablespoons lime juice
1 tablespoon chopped fresh cilantro

1 tablespoon chopped green onions
1 to 2 tablespoons chopped jalapeño
   peppers (2 to 3 medium)
½ teaspoon garlic salt

Combine all ingredients; mix well. Cover and refrigerate at least one hour. Makes 6 (½-cup) servings.
Source: National Watermelon Promotion Board

August 8   Not Just for Bones!

Nearly everyone knows that calcium keeps bones healthy at every age. Today's science is revealing more. Eating enough calcium may:

- *Lower colon cancer risk,* likely by counteracting the effects of high-fat eating.
- *Help reduce blood pressure* (along with potassium and magnesium) among sodium-sensitive people. (No test exists yet to know who's sodium sensitive.)

Early research suggests that consuming enough calcium *may* be linked to: less chance of kidney stones, and—if calcium comes from food—less discomfort from PMS symptoms for some, protection from polycystic ovary syndrome, less obesity risk since calcium may discourage body fat deposits, and perhaps lower risk of insulin resistance syndrome and the start of diabetes.

The recommended amount is 1,000 milligrams of calcium daily for younger adults; 1,200 milligrams daily after age 50.

For enough calcium:

- *Get it from food, the best source.* Dairy foods (milk, yogurt, cheese) have the most, then perhaps calcium-fortified foods (soy beverages, juice, cereal), followed by fish with edible bones, and some greens.
- *Take a calcium supplement if you need more.* Calcium phosphate, calcium citrate, or calcium gluconate are absorbed better than calcium carbonate or oyster shell calcium.

August 9   Spin Doctor

When did you last ride a bike? Fortunately, bike riding is one skill you probably won't forget. So dust off your own bike or borrow one from a teen, and start pedaling!

Pumping your legs pumps your heart muscle for a heart-healthy workout. Even bicycling at less than 10 miles an hour burns 220 calories per hour if you weigh 120 pounds, and 310 calories per hour if you weigh 170. Your leg muscles get stronger, especially pedaling uphill. And you can do it in your own neighborhood, with your family.

Go for a spin today.

- *Bike around your neighborhood.* Try for 30 minutes daily.
- *Ride for practicality.* Take your bike, not your car, on a nearby errand or to visit friends.
- *Join a spinning class at a local fitness club.* You'll ride a stationery bike.

August 10   Flax Facts

Flax: For thousands of years, this blue-flowering crop has been cultivated for food, linen cloth, and fine-quality paper. Today we're learning *why* flaxseeds are good for you.

Let's start with taste: Flaxseeds add a nutty flavor to breads, muffins, cookies, cereal bars, pancakes, even smoothies! Buy flaxseeds whole, ground, or as flour.

As for health: Small, oil-rich flaxseeds are high in *omega-3* fatty acids. Omega-3s may help lower your heart disease risk, protect you from heart arrhythmia, and boost your immune system.

Flaxseed contains two types of *fiber:* soluble, with cholesterol-lowering properties, and insoluble, with potential cancer-fighting ability. Flaxseed is also rich in *lignan* (phytoestrogen), which may help protect against breast and prostate cancers.

Cook with flaxseed.

- *Get in the grind.* For health benefits, grind whole flaxseeds in a coffee grinder until granular or processed into flour. In a recipe flax can replace some flour.
- *Use flaxseeds as a fat replacer.* If a recipe calls for ⅓ cup oil or shortening, use 1 cup of milled flaxseed instead. When flaxseed replaces oil, baked goods tend to brown faster.
- *Another nutri-bit:* Omega-3-enriched eggs come from hens that eat flaxseed.

August 11   Passport to Health—Eating India Style

Curry, turmeric, other spices, chutney, more! These seasonings flavor the cuisine of India, giving distinction to lentils, rice, vegetables, and other plant-based dishes.

If you pick a restaurant featuring Indian cuisine, enjoy the many combinations with plant-based ingredients: baked roti, lentil dishes, vegetable dishes made with yogurt, chicken or fish dishes with vegetable sauces, or naan. Go easy on curry dishes made with coconut milk, fried bread (poori, paratha), and fried samosas; their fat and calories add up.

Prepare a simple India-inspired dish yourself.

- *Find an easy curry recipe.* Check in a vegetarian magazine or cookbook.
- *Switch to basmati rice.* With its fragrant, nutty flavor, it's great in any recipe that calls for long-grain rice.
- *Flavor with chutney.* Accent rice, grilled chicken, and broiled fish with this piquant relish.

Raisin Apricot Chutney

½ cup raisins
½ cup chopped dried apricots
2 tablespoons chopped onion
1½ cups apple juice
3 tablespoons cider vinegar

3 tablespoons brown sugar
2 tablespoons chopped crystallized
  ginger
½ teaspoon ground cloves

Combine raisins, apricots, onion, and apple juice in medium saucepan. Cook over low heat 20 minutes or until apricots and raisins are plump and tender, stirring occasionally. Add vinegar, brown sugar, ginger, and cloves. Bring to a boil. Cook and stir until sugar is dissolved. Refrigerate 8 hours or more to blend flavors. Makes 5 (¼-cup) servings.

Source: California Raisin Marketing Board

August 12 Taste the Difference?

Do spicy foods taste especially hot? Do bitter or tart flavors make you wince? If so, you may be a supertaster. With more papillae, you taste more intensely.

Fact is, we do taste the same foods differently. Age and genes affect how many taste buds (found in papillae) we have on our tongue, throat, and mouth lining. Kids have more; older adults, less. Health problems may also diminish sensory ability. Because we eat foods that taste good to us, taste perception affects our food choices, nutrition, even health.

Whether you're a supertaster or not, prepare food well; enjoy it at its peak freshness for the most flavor. Savor food slowly; chew well to release food's full taste, aroma, and mouth feel. Eat a variety of foods to stimulate your taste buds. (*Tip:* Your senses are more acute when you're hungry.)

Are you a supertaster?

- With a hole puncher, punch a hole in a small piece of wax paper.
- Put the hole on the tip of your tongue; wipe it with blue food coloring.
- With a mirror, magnifying glass, and flashlight, count the papillae. Nontasters only have five or six; supertasters have dozens of them!

August 13 Eating Single-Handed

Got the phone, the steering wheel, or your computer mouse in one hand—and food in the other? Two-handed eating, when you're relaxed and focused on food and your body's fullness cues, may be healthier. By paying attention, you're less likely to overeat.

If you're trying to eat and drive, pull over. It's safer, less messy, and gives you a chance for a brisk walk to stretch your legs.

That said, if you need "portafuel," make it nutrient-rich instead of grabbing a bag of chips, a candy bar, or a hefty to-go burger.

- *From the deli:* wrap sandwich, sushi, sub sandwich, fruit smoothie (Whatever your choice, be sensible with portion size.)
- *From the drive-thru:* grilled chicken sandwich, regular-size burger (not deluxe-size), cup of cut-up fruit, carton of milk or juice
- *From the bakery:* warm pretzel, bagel (go easy on the cream cheese), latte or chai
- *From the supermarket:* baby carrots, whole fruit, small package of nuts or dried fruit, can of juice, milk

August 14 Move More, Live Longer

Inactivity is a big health threat, perhaps accounting for 2.5 million deaths over the next decade. Labeled as Sedentary Death Syndrome (SeDS), inactivity has health risks beyond obesity.

Staying active can downsize your risks of chronic disease.

- *Heart health.* Regular aerobic exercise boosts HDL- (good) cholesterol, may slow atherosclerosis, and may help control blood pressure.
- *Bone health.* Both weight-bearing activity and the push and pull of muscles with bones help keep bones strong by stimulating calcium deposits.
- *Protection from diabetes.* By improving glucose metabolism, being active may help protect against type 2 diabetes.

- *Cancer protection.* Regular activity also reduces some cancer risk.
- *Brain function.* Regular activity may promote memory, learning, and thinking skills—and maybe lower the chances of dementia, mental decline, and Alzheimer's disease.

Move more to increase your chances for a longer, healthier life.

- *Spend at least 15 minutes more doing something active (anything!) today*—it doesn't need to be sports.
- *Write down three ways to add 15 minutes of active living every-day*—until you move 60 minutes daily.

August 15   Cook Savvy—In the Sub-Way

Easy kitchen tip? Cut calories when you cook today by barely changing your recipe. Just make a simple substitution or two.

If a recipe calls for . . .	Use . . .	Saved in recipe calories (rounded)
½ cup sour cream	½ cup regular plain yogurt	140
	½ cup low-fat cottage cheese with 1½ teaspoons lemon juice	125
½ cup cream	½ cup evaporated fat-free milk	195
1 cup part-skim ricotta cheese	1 cup low-fat cottage cheese	180
½ cup mayonnaise	¼ cup regular plain yogurt *plus* ¼ cup low-fat cottage cheese	725
¼ pound bacon	¼ pound lean ham	480
1 pound regular ground beef	1 pound extra-lean ground beef	115
1 egg (as thickener)	1 tablespoon flour	45
1 egg yolk (large)	1 egg white (large)	45
1 cup oil in muffin or quick bread batter	½ cup puréed fruit (sweetened applesauce) *plus* ½ cup oil	895
1 cup sweetened, shredded coconut	½ cup toasted, sweetened, shredded coconut *plus* ½ teaspoon coconut extract	150

August 16   🌾 Figure Your Future

Wonder what size jeans you'll wear 10 years from now? Even if your weight is healthy today, the way that you eat now may foretell your weight in another decade, notes a Boston University 12-year study of 700 women.

Try to predict your future figure. Are you a . . .

☐ *Heart-Healthy Eater:* more nutrient-dense fruits and vegetables, and lean food servings with less fat, saturated fat, and cholesterol, and more carbohydrate and fiber

☐ *Light Eater:* fewer calories, but more fat and saturated fat than a Heart-Healthy eater

☐ *Moderate Eater:* moderate eating

☐ *High-Fat Eater:* more animal and vegetable fats, sweets and desserts, meats, sodas, and other sweetened beverages

☐ *Empty-Calorie Eater:* similar to a High-Fat Eater

Over time, suggests the study, heart-healthy eating, followed by light eating, may be your best bet to keep pounds off. Light eating also was linked to more weight fluctuation. Not surprisingly, high-fat and empty-calorie eating seem to increase the chance of becoming overweight.

To wear the jeans that match your healthy weight:

• *Review the food-group guidelines* (from January 15 and 16) to help you choose varied, moderate amounts of mostly lean and low-fat foods. It's the best heart-healthy weight control guide around.

August 17   🍎 Spread Health Benefits

Are you among the nearly 100 million or so Americans with higher than normal blood cholesterol? If so, a butterlike spread made with plant stanol or sterol esters may help bring your LDL- (bad) cholesterol down, without affecting your HDL- (good) cholesterol level.

Plant stanol and sterol esters, also found naturally in small amounts in vegetables and plant oils, help block cholesterol in the intestine from being absorbed. That helps lower LDL-cholesterol in the bloodstream.

Anyone can get the cholesterol-lowering benefits, but people with high blood cholesterol levels get more. For the record, these spreads are safe to use if you are taking cholesterol-lowering statin drugs.

If your LDL-cholesterol is higher than normal:

- *Ask your physician about using these spreads* with plant sterols or stanol esters, sold as Take Control and Benecol.
- *Use them according to package directions*—two to three servings daily with meals—as a butter or margarine substitute.
- *Follow cholesterol-lowering advice, too:* eat a diet low in saturated fat and cholesterol, stay physically active, and eat plenty of fruit, vegetables, and whole-grain breads and cereals.

August 18   Today Is Play Day!

Remember when you ran through the sprinkler on a hot summer day, played Frisbee with a frolicking pet, or ran simply for the joy of it? Bring out your playfulness, and enjoy the mental and physical health benefits.

Research shows that most children stay active into their 'tweens. After that, activity levels decline sharply as active playtime turns into sedentary teenage leisure. Once people launch their adult lives, physical activity competes with busy living. The result: a sedentary lifestyle as a risk factor for many health problems.

Wind up your summer with active play.

- *Play actively with kids.* Play tag, jump rope, or hide-and-seek.
- *Take a vacation day to play.* It's good for your head!
- *Feel free to move with the childlike spirit of youth.* With that mental outlook, you'll stay healthier and feel younger, too.

August 19   Through the Grapevine

Looking for an easy, low-calorie, yet sweet snack? Grab a handful of grapes now, during peak season. So easy: no preparation—just wash them under cold water.

Nutritionally speaking, grapes supply *vitamin C,* but less than other fruit. Depending on their variety, they have varying amounts of *flavonoids: resveratrol, quercetin, anthocyanins,* and *catechins.* Found mainly in the skin, resveratrol in grapes may help reduce heart disease risk. Early research suggests a role in cancer protection, too.

Refresh your palate with grapes today.

- *Toss halved grapes in salad*—spinach salad, slaw, pasta salad, or chicken or seafood salad. Make it portable as a salad wrap.
- *Freeze grapes*—a refreshing snack, or can be used as "ice cubes" in water, iced tea, or fruit juice.

Tropical Fruit Salad

2 cups seedless grapes
1 medium banana, peeled and sliced
1 mango, peeled and cubed
1 teaspoon grated fresh ginger
½ cup low-fat tropical fruit–flavored yogurt
4 mint sprigs

Combine grapes, banana, and mango; toss to mix. Stir ginger into yogurt. Spoon dressing over mixed fruits, or add to fruits and mix to combine. Portion into individual glass bowls; garnish with mint. Makes 4 servings.
Source: California Table Grape Commission

August 20   Catch the News Today

Was there a "startling" headline with the "latest" nutrition research? Take heed before accepting it as new advice. Even results from well-devised research aren't necessarily facts—and may not apply to you.

In the past, health professionals had time to interpret study findings and come to scientific consensus before research became public knowledge. Health experts still do this. But media, mostly less qualified to interpret science, may tell the story sooner, in sound bites, without reflecting the whole picture or the limits or extent of the study.

To judge whether a study is credible and relevant to you:

- *Read the bottom line.* Perspectives from qualified experts may appear at the story's end.
- *Look for replication.* One or two studies aren't enough.
- *Check for a human dimension.* Animal studies are first steps, not always relevant to people.
- *See if it applies to you.* Data from subjects like you is likely more relevant for you. Studies done only on men may not apply to women and vice versa. Ask your doctor.
- *Keep a healthy skepticism.* Qualified nutrition experts offer advice only when there's enough scientific consensus.
- *Get an expert opinion.* A registered dietitian can help judge the report and put the findings in context for you. Check the American Dietetic Association's Web site for a local expert: www.eatright.org.

August 21   Another Fishy Story

Buying fish for dinner? These clues can help you judge its freshness and safety:

- *Fresh fish fillets and steaks:* mild scent; firm, moist flesh; translucent appearance; no browning around the edges; if wrapped, tight undamaged packaging
- *Fresh, whole finfish:* ocean-breeze scent; firm to the touch; stiff fins; tight scales; shiny-"metallic" skin; pink to bright-red gills; clear, bright, protruding eyes
- *Shellfish:* mild aroma for raw shrimp; scallops that aren't dry or dark around the edges. Unless cooked, frozen, or canned, clams, mussels, and oysters in their shell should be alive, with slightly open shells that close when tapped.
- *Frozen fish and frozen-prepared fish items:* frozen sold; mild odor; free of ice crystals and freezer burn
- *Cooked shellfish:* moist, mild odor; characteristic color (e.g., pink to reddish shells on shrimp, bright-red for lobsters, crabs, and crayfish)

For safety, avoid buying cooked fish displayed next to raw fish. When you shop for fish:

- *Go easy on breaded shrimp and fish sticks,* which have more fat and calories.
- *Fresh fish.* Buy just what you'll eat right away.
- *Stock for convenience:* canned salmon, tuna, or mackerel, or frozen shrimp or fish fillets or steaks.

August 22   Caution—Herbals

True or false? Since they're "natural," herbals are safe and effective. *False.* Herbal supplements are neither well tested nor well regulated. "Natural" doesn't mean "effective," "mild effect," or "safe" as you may use them. Some herbals may be more harmful than healthful!

A lot of unknowns surround herbal supplements and their use. We don't know all their bioactive substances and what they do, how different varieties of the same herbal compare, how growing conditions affect their bioactive substances, how substances in one herbal interact with another or with food or medication, how much is effective or harmful. They aren't tested or regulated as medicines are.

If you take an herbal supplement, be cautious!

- *Learn about its risks and possible side effects first.* It may be especially dangerous to take if you have health problems.
- *Get your doctor's okay, talk to your pharmacist.* Herbals aren't advised for women who are pregnant, trying to become pregnant, or breastfeeding, or for children.
- *Use only as directed.* An herbal can be toxic in high doses, taken for a long time, or combined with other supplements or medications.
- *Avoid herbals*—if you're on medication since they may interfere with drug action, if you're going in for surgery, if you feel side effects, or if they offer no benefits.

August 23   Get Fresh

Unopened packaged foods: is what's inside fresh? Read the label! Many have dates you can read:

- *"Best if used by" date:* not a safety date, but when the food is at top quality
- *Pack date:* when the food was manufactured, processed, or packaged
- *"Sell by" date:* last date a food should be sold so it's fresh for home storage
- *Julian date (on eggs):* a number between 001 (January 1) and 365 (December 31) that shows when eggs are packed. Refrigerated eggs keep their quality for four to five weeks after that.

Some packaged and canned foods carry a letter or number code you can't interpret. Contact the food company to learn the manufacturing date and what the code means.

During these lazy summer days, clean your kitchen—and keep your stock of packaged foods fresh.

- *Rotate: first in, first out.* Put the newest items toward the back of the fridge, freezer, or cabinet.
- *Toss food that's been around too long.* Spoiled food may not have a bad aroma. Never taste to check.
- *Wonder about unopened canned foods?* They keep their best quality for about two years. After that, they're still safe to use if the seal is intact and the can isn't bulging.
- *Clean your refrigerator.* It runs more efficiently; it's easier to organize, and it's safer.

August 24 🏥 Headache Prone?

Project deadlines, airport delays, cranky kids—what gives *you* a tension headache?

Millions of people suffer from chronic headaches—sometimes debilitating migraines—that don't go away easily. Many blame certain foods. But the causes are more complicated and not well understood. Food's effect is likely small. It may trigger a headache only when combined with something else, perhaps stress, medication, weather changes, a hormone change, or some physical activities. Among suspected yet unproven food triggers: tyrosine (in coffee and chocolate), histamine (in red wine), caffeine (in coffee, chocolate, and cola), nitrates (in luncheon meats and hot dogs), benzoic acid (a preservative), and alcohol.

Ice cream headaches? That happens if an area in the roof of your mouth gets cold fast, affecting nerve endings that trigger headaches. Although intense, they don't last long—thankfully.

Prone to headaches, and not sure why?

- *Keep a headache diary.* For a week, track the time and date, intensity, other symptoms, medications and dosage, and possible triggers (food, weather, stressors, fatigue level, physical activity). For women, keep track of menstrual cycles, too. Suspect a food? Try it again later. See what happens.
- *Learn how to relieve stress.* Read April 15 and May 22.
- *Limit caffeine if it's a problem.* Cut back slowly; consuming less caffeine can cause headaches as your body adjusts.
- *Drink enough fluids.* Dehydration can trigger headaches.
- *Check with your doctor to rule out other causes.* If you get food-related migraines, talk to a registered dietitian for food substitutions.

August 25   Wrap It Up for Health

Want an easy hand-held meal? Just wrap and roll nourishing, flavorful ingredients in a tortilla or flat bread.

- *Start with a sturdy, pliable wheat tortilla or flat bread.* Try tomato, spinach, or other flavored tortillas.
- *Layer on well-dried greens:* lettuce, spinach, watercress, other greens.
- *Spread on cooked grains:* bulgur, couscous, rice (or tabouli; see May 14).
- *Flavor with salsa or salad dressing.* Go easy so the filling won't be soggy.
- *Add crunchy veggies:* diced bell peppers, onion, mushrooms, sprouts, drained canned beans.
- *Top with meat, chicken, or seafood (optional).* Slice it first.
- *Fold in the ends; roll!*

Ordering out? Wraps aren't necessarily low-fat or low-calorie. A high-fat sauce or dressing, or a wrap that's twice what you need, may supply enough extra calories or fat for two meals.

Wrap leftovers or "plan-overs" for a quick lunch or supper.

Southwest Tortilla Wraps

2 tablespoons low-fat salad dressing or mayonnaise	½ cup thin strips red pepper
4 10-inch flour tortillas	¼ cup sliced green onions
½ cup chunky salsa	2 tablespoons sliced black olives
4 ounces sliced turkey or roast beef	pinch of cayenne pepper, optional
⅓ cup shredded low-fat Cheddar cheese	

Spread salad dressing on tortillas; spread salsa over salad dressing. Top with turkey or meat, cheese, vegetables, and cayenne pepper as desired. Roll and serve, or heat 45 seconds in microwave oven on medium power. Each tortilla can be wrapped in plastic wrap after rolling and then refrigerated. Makes 4 servings.
Source: Wheat Foods Council

August 26 On a Whim

Surprised when the cash register totals up a grocery bill that far exceeds your budget? Maybe you're an impulse shopper. And you may bring home foods you don't use, need, or ultimately eat.

If you grocery shop today:

- *Plan ahead.* Make a shopping list and stick to it.
- *Snack beforehand.* Or drink bottled water for a temporary full feeling. Studies show that hungry people buy more.
- *Steer your cart away from sampling tables.* If you do taste, buy only if you really want it, not because a taste feels like an obligation.
- *Size up food displays.* Before grabbing attention-catching foods or drinks, decide if you really want them, even at a price saving.

August 27 Necessity—Mother of Invention

Can you identify these historical figures: Percy Spencer, Nicolas Appert, Luther Burbank, or Fanny Farmer? Maybe not, but their work likely affects what you eat nearly every day. Spencer invented the microwave oven (1946); Appert, the canning process (1770s); Burbank developed the Idaho potato (1871) and many popular varieties of potatoes, plums, and berries; Farmer, standard cooking measurements (published, 1896).

August is National Inventors Month, a good time to honor how America's inventiveness has brought more nutrition, better food safety, and more food choices to your table.

Among the inventions of the last century: vitamin D–fortified milk, iron-enriched flour, and folic acid–fortified grain products. Today scientists are developing tomatoes with more cancer-protecting lycopene, peanuts with less of the protein that causes allergic reactions, higher-starch potatoes that absorb less fat for chips and fries, among others.

Reinvent your food choices this month.

- *Invent one solution to a personal eating challenge.* Here's one: Spoon cut-up fruit into an unsugared ice cream cone to eat on the run.
- *Invent a new dish.* Just change one ingredient: fennel or kohlrabi in soups or stir-fries, or atemoya or blood orange in fruit salads.

August 28   Forget It, Okay?

Do your glasses, keys, or shoes hide? Need to jot things down so you don't forget? Short memory lapses probably aren't a first sign of Alzheimer's. More likely, it's normal aging. You lose neuron-to-neuron links even in young adulthood. But if you have a family history of Alzheimer's, talk to your physician.

Can nutrition help prevent forgetful moments? Perhaps, but so far research can't offer definitive advice. Some B vitamins may play a role. Experts advise B vitamin–rich foods, not supplements: green leafy vegetables, legumes, grain foods, milk, meat, and fortified breads and cereals. Antioxidant-rich fruits and vegetables may help keep nerve cells healthy. As for ginkgo biloba for healthy people, there's not enough reliable research to know if it helps.

To keep mentally sharp as you age:

- *Do mental gymnastics.* Read a challenging book. Add numbers mentally. Unfamiliar tasks and new ways of thinking may develop underused brain connections.
- *Eat smarter.* Nourish your brain with nutrient-rich foods.
- *Manage your health.* Any health problem that disrupts blood flow to your brain affects thinking and memory. That includes diabetes, heart disease, and high blood pressure.
- *Stay physically active; fit in aerobic activity.* That keeps blood vessels open so oxygen gets to the brain for normal function.
- *Sleep enough; reduce stress.* A memory lapse may really be fatigue or disorganization!

August 29 Fit or Fat?

Watching your weight? Your bathroom scale won't tell the whole story. After all, muscle weighs more than body fat. Although body composition helps define fitness, a typical bathroom scale can't differentiate body fat from muscle weight.

Tip: If you're trying to lose weight, be physically active to build muscle as you eat fewer calories. Then you won't lose muscle. If you're trying to gain weight, work out so you gain muscle, not just body fat.

What % Body Fat Is Healthy?

	18 to 39 Years	40 to 59 Years	60 to 79 Years
Females	21–32%	23–33%	24–35%
Males	8–19%	11–21%	13–24%

Source: Shape Up America, www.shapeup.org/bodylab/frmst.htm

Body fat is measured in several ways, among them with skin calipers to measure the fat layer in several places under the skin and with bioelectrical impedance analysis (BIA) that uses a low-level electrical signal, passing through muscle and fat (slower through muscle).

To have your body fat measured accurately:

- *Ask at your next medical checkup.*
- *Check with a certified trainer,* if you belong to a fitness club with well-trained staff.
- *Get a well-rated body fat scale,* one that not only weighs you but also gives a BIA. Learn to use it with accuracy: same time of day (midday best), same settings, after urinating.

August 30 Cravings—In Your Head

Ever feel like you *must* have a bag of chips, a chocolate bar, a spoon-ful of peanut butter? Cravings are normal. Their causes aren't clear—psychological, physical, or both. Perhaps your body craves foods with nutrients you need. Or maybe positive emotions, memories, and social situations reinforce your food cravings.

Should you give in to a craving, especially if it's not a fruit or veg-etable? Sure, now and then, if most of your food choices are nutrient-rich and if you keep portions small. Being rigid isn't healthy.

To tame a craving:

- *Find a distraction.* With the immediate stimulus gone, your craving may disappear, too. If you still want it later, have a small portion.
- *Pick a better-for-you version:* perhaps frozen yogurt instead of premium ice cream for less fat and more calcium.
- *Have a small taste.* Being overly restrictive can make food irre-sistible. Then guilt creeps in, too!
- *Listen to your body cues.* Maybe hunger triggered a craving.
- *Know what triggers your craving:* perhaps chocolates in easy sight or the aroma of popcorn as you walk through the mall. Avoid it!
- *Brush your teeth; gargle with mouthwash.* That may extinguish your craving.
- *Plan ahead.* Have a small amount of another food handy, per-haps carrot sticks or pretzels.

August 31   🛒 What's on Tap?

Tap water or bottled? Your choice. You might like bottled water for convenience or for what it doesn't have: sugar, calories, caffeine, or alcohol. But it costs 240 to 10,000 times more per gallon than tap water, which has the same benefits!

In the United States, either bottled or tap water is safe from bacteria. For tap water, that's especially true if it's from a large municipal water system. Since tap water is chlorine treated, you might prefer a bottled-water taste.

Is your tap water "hard" (with minerals)? If you don't like its slightly metallic taste, consider a filter. The most effective ones meet this standard: National Sanitation Foundation International Standard 53.

One safety issue to consider is excessive lead from water pipes in older homes. If you're concerned, ask your water utility company to test it. *Note:* most tap water is fluoridated, important for kids' oral health; bottled water usually isn't.

During August, National Water Quality Month:

- *Store a safe water supply for an emergency.* Figure one gallon a day per person. Buy gallon jugs of water, or store tap water in clean food-quality containers—not reused milk jugs. Date each container. Keep them in a cool, dry, dark place. Change them every six months. Read May 12 again.
- *Wash water bottles*—in hot, soapy water. Not only your "sports bottle," but also your empty bottled water bottle if it's reused. Sipping the same bottle of water over several days contaminates it with bacteria.

September 1   🩺 Protein Mania?

Need more protein, less carbohydrate for weight control? More likely, you need fewer calories in (from food) and more calories out (from active living). Consider:

- *Quick weight loss from high-protein eating often comes from water loss.* Possible side effects are dehydration, constipation, and strain on the kidneys.
- *High-carb foods in a varied meal won't make you hungrier.* Well-chosen high-carb, fiber-rich vegetables, fruits, legumes (beans), and whole-grain food choices help you feel full. That promotes weight loss and reduces major chronic disease risk.
- *Eating carbohydrate-rich foods doesn't cause insulin resistance that makes people fat.* Obesity, inactivity, aging, and perhaps genetics are the real issues related to insulin resistance.
- *No evidence shows that excess carb calories become body fat more easily than calories from fat.*
- *Most Americans under age 65 already eat considerably more protein than needed.*
- *To add to the confusion, there's no one definition of a high-protein diet.*

Note: No long-term clinical studies show sustained benefits from high-protein weight-loss diets.

If you're considering a weight-loss approach:

- *Get carbs from high-fiber foods:* Fiber-rich whole-grain foods, beans, vegetables, and fruits will help you feel full.
- *Eat for variety; keep portions sensible.* Bottom line: Eat nutrient-rich foods but consume fewer calories.
- *Be physically active*—at least 60 minutes of moderate activity daily.
- *Still want a high-protein diet?* Follow it for just a short time. Then switch to more-balanced eating.

September 2   Energy—Worth Saving?

Leaf blowers and self-cleaning ovens, garage door openers and car washes. Just think of all the labor-saving devices that make your life easier—and more sedentary than ever!

By spending these "labor savings" on walking, bike riding, or other physical activities, you *could* burn that same amount of energy (calories) you saved and net out even. But do you? On average, Americans spend 500 calories less per day than they did 50 years ago, which contributes to today's increasing obesity rates.

Skip labor savers this Labor Day Weekend. Get the health benefits of moving more.

- *Wash and wax your own car for an hour.* Spend 280 more calories than using the car wash.
- *Rake your leaves.* Spend 50 calories more for each half hour than with a leaf blower. (Avoids noise pollution, too!)
- *Shop at the mall.* Spend 210 calories more per hour by mall walking than with online shopping.

September 3   Beat the Breakfast Blahs

In a breakfast rut? Do you mindlessly pour breakfast cereal and milk into a bowl? That's okay—as long as you make a nutritious morning meal part of your morning routine.

In fact, a morning meal is well known to boost productivity and concentration and, for kids, to be important for learning. And because breakfast takes the edge off morning hunger and deters late-morning nibbling, studies show that breakfast is a great strategy for weight control, too.

To celebrate Better Breakfast Month, think out of the cereal box.

- *Toasted waffle sandwich:* toasted freezer waffles, filled with lean ham, Cheddar shreds, and apple or tomato slices
- *Fresh breakfast salad:* greens tossed with chopped Canadian bacon, chopped pecans, and maple syrup vinaigrette (apple cider vinegar, oil, and a splash of maple syrup), then topped with toast croutons
- *Breakfast in a cup:* chopped seasonal fruit, topped with yogurt and granola, in a plastic "to go" cup

September 4   Energy Slump?

Before you blame your midday energy dip on low blood sugar, take note. Unless you have diabetes, hypoglycemia is far less common than once thought. Slumps may come from the normal release of the hormone epinephrine.

For those without diabetes, some conditions boost the chance of hypoglycemia: long, strenuous exercise; prolonged fasting; early stages of pregnancy; drinking alcoholic beverages; or taking beta blockers for those who exercise.

In rare cases, people experience reactive hypoglycemia two to five hours after eating a large meal; their body secretes too much insulin so blood sugar drops well below normal.

Before you self-diagnose hypoglycemia:

- *Check with your physician.* Have a reliable test *while* you experience the symptoms. Be aware: similar symptoms may come from health conditions unrelated to blood sugar. If you truly have hypoglycemia, seek advice from a registered dietitian.
- *Eat healthfully, exercise regularly, live smart.* Make sure your symptoms aren't confused with extreme hunger or fatigue from poor lifestyle habits.

September 5   Clucking About the Benefits

Looking for something nutritious, economical, and easy to cook? Grilled or stir-fried, roasted or braised, chicken's a healthful choice for your family meal.

A great *protein* source, chicken is also low in total fat, saturated fat, and cholesterol, especially without the skin. (Most sat fats are in the skin.) Three ounces of cooked skinless chicken breast have 4.5 grams of fat and 1.5 grams of saturated fat. Breast or leg: both are healthful. The breast has a little less fat. But dark meat (leg) has more iron (and more flavor), and less fat and sat fat than many meat cuts.

To keep chicken moist, tender, and flavorful, cook it "skin on." A thin membrane between the skin and the flesh keeps moisture in and fat out of the flesh. Just remove the skin before eating, and halve the fat content.

During National Chicken Month, plan a quick, flavorful chicken dinner tonight.

- *Cook chicken legs on the grill.* Slather with your favorite barbecue sauce.
- *In a rush? Buy precooked chicken strips or chunks*—great for quick salads, sandwiches, pizza toppers, tortilla stuffers.
- *Roast a whole chicken.* Fill the cavity with sliced lemon, onion, and fresh rosemary before roasting.

September 6   Rice—Always Nice

Do you toss "factoids" into party talk? Here's one for National Rice Month: the world grows more than 40,000 types of rice and about 1.3 trillion pounds of rice annually—a lot of rice!

Store shelves may display more than traditional white rice: arborio (short-grain for risotto); aromatic, often nutty-flavored rices (Basmati, Black Japonica, jasmine, Texmati, Wehani); brown rices (all whole-grain), among others.

Good for you? You bet! Any rice is high in complex carbs. Enriched white rice has thiamin, niacin, folic acid, and iron added. Brown rice offers these nutrients, and with its bran layer intact, even more fiber and protein, too.

Enjoy rice—in soup or salad, or perhaps in pilaf, paella, risotto, or stir-fried rice.

Red Bean and Rice Salad with Mango

2   cups cooked brown rice
1   15-ounce can red kidney beans, drained and rinsed
¾ cup finely chopped green bell pepper
½ cup fresh mango, cut in ½-inch pieces
½ cup finely chopped red onion
½ cup salsa, drained
salt and freshly ground pepper to taste
2   tablespoons chopped fresh cilantro

In a large bowl, combine rice, beans, pepper, mango, and onion. Add drained salsa and mix into salad. Season to taste with salt and pepper. Just before serving, sprinkle with cilantro. Makes 4 servings.

Source: American Institute for Cancer Research

September 7   Home Work—Eat Smart

Whether paid work or volunteer work, working at home offers easy kitchen access. Whether that's a benefit or a hazard to smart eating depends on you.

To eat smart as a home-office habit, set regular mealtimes, rather than heading to the kitchen on a break. When you do need a break, "do" rather than eat: walk the dog, pick a flower bouquet, start a laundry load. Especially if you work alone, go out for an occasional lunch with a friend or a colleague. Enjoy the home-office advantage: take your afternoon break to put dinner in the oven or start a simmering pot of hearty stew.

Since you likely have no workplace deli or cafeteria to rely on:

- *Stock your kitchen for easy workday meals:* fruit, canned soups and stews, salad ingredients, whole-grain bread, lean deli meat and cheese, frozen microwave "bowls" and other prepared foods, milk, yogurt.
- *Plan ahead, then re-create last night's leftovers.* Heat leftover stir-fries, and wrap in a warm tortilla for a quick fajita. Microwave a baked potato; top with yesterday's stew or lentil soup. Slice leftover chicken to arrange on a freshly tossed salad.

September 8   Tailgating 101

Summer's on the wane. Soon cool, crisp autumn air and a colorful landscape add seasonal flair to tailgate parties at parking lots, fields, and roadsides. This season make yours . . .

- *Safe.* Even with a chill in the air, remember picnic food safety. Keep perishables in a clean, well-chilled cooler until mealtime, and during the game if you plan to eat afterward. Wrap hot dishes in several layers of newspaper, or in an insulated heat-and-tote container; eat them right away at the tailgate site. Toss leftovers that sit out longer than an hour or so. Pack an antibacterial handwash to use after handling meat, poultry, fish, or any food. (See May 25 and July 7.)

- *Healthful:* Pack a thermos of hot cider, cocoa, or soup. Bring pretzels, crisp veggies and salsa, and crunchy fall apples; go easy on fried pork rinds, chips, and dips. Barbecue chicken breasts, shrimp kebobs, or lean meats on the spot!
- *Active:* Bring a ball or Frisbee to toss around.

For easy, flavorful complements in tailgate meals:

- *Grill vegetables*: sliced eggplant, bell pepper, sweet potato, brushed lightly with oil. Great hot or cold.
- *Make a multibean salad* with any combination of three or more canned beans and low-fat Italian dressing.
- *Assemble antipasto.* Surround precooked, whole-grain couscous with canned artichokes, hearts of palm, roasted peppers, garbanzos, sliced tomatoes, blanched green beans or asparagus. Drizzle with vinaigrette.

September 9 Cooks on the Move

Ever think of cooking as an active sport? TV chefs are in constant motion: chopping, stirring, whisking, scrubbing, lifting—physically multitasking!

Join the kitchen team whenever you can. It takes more muscle, more motion, and more energy to prepare food from scratch than to simply pop a prepared meal into the microwave oven.

Join in some culinary athletics.

- *Knead a batch of homemade dough*—great for your arm and shoulder muscles.
- *Whip egg whites, batter, and mashed potatoes by hand*—good for arm muscles.
- *Tromp through farmer's markets.* Walking and carrying bags of produce are good weight-bearing activities.
- *Pick tree fruit at a local grove*—great stretching, and hauling fruit to your car builds muscles.

September 10   Hi Ho, the Dairy Oh

At any age, you need the nutrition benefits that milk supplies. But which milk for you? And what if you're a strict vegetarian? You have plenty of choices in the dairy case.

- *Fat-free, low-fat, reduced-fat, or whole milk.* No matter what type, 8 ounces (1 cup) has about 300 milligrams of calcium, along with protein, riboflavin, vitamins A and D, phosphorus, and other vitamins and minerals. The difference is their fat and calorie content: for 1 cup, from 85 calories and less than 1 fat gram in fat-free milk to 150 calories and 8 fat grams in whole milk.
- *Flavored milk.* Chocolate, fruit, or other flavors—it has all the nutrients of unflavored milk. Check the label to see if it's vitamin D fortified.
- *Acidophilus milk.* Processed with "friendly" bacteria, it's usually made from low-fat or fat-free milk. Benefit? It may improve lactose digestion and promote a healthy intestinal tract.
- *Lactose-free or lactose-reduced milk.* It's treated with a lactase enzyme, so it's easier to digest if you're lactose intolerant.
- *Soy beverages.* They don't have all the nutrients of cows' milk, but they may be fortified with calcium, vitamins A and D, and riboflavin; check the label. Soy drinks range from 80 to 500 milligrams calcium per cup. Choose one with more calcium, since calcium in soy beverages isn't absorbed as well as from cow's milk.

Drink your choice of milk today.

- *Mix in iced latte or chai.*
- *Swirl in a fruit-dairy smoothie.*
- *Buy a carton with your fast-food burger.*
- *Use in creamy soups to make them "creamier."*

September 11 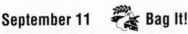 Bag It!

Imagine your alarm goes off. You stretch, then race to get ready for the day. How will you pack your family's lunches?

During back-to-school, back-to-work season, get creative with healthful pack-and-go lunches.

- *Hand-y.* Finger foods are easy to eat: sandwiches, wraps, pita pockets. Go beyond sandwiches: soft pretzels, string cheese, or hummus with veggie sticks.
- *Crunch in your lunch.* Tuck in crisp raw vegetables (peppers, celery, carrots, zucchini, broccoli), fresh fruit (tangerine, apple, grapes, pear), whole-grain foods (crackers, popcorn, pretzels), and nuts.
- *Add some fun:* baked chips, oatmeal cookies, trail mix.
- *Heaviest on the bottom.* Pack juice cans, whole fruit, yogurt, pudding cups, and other heavy items on the bottom so they don't crush other foods.
- *Chill out.* Use an insulated bag with cold packs to keep food cold and safe. Freeze juice or bottled water for double duty: chilling and drinking. (No need to rely on vending machine soda.)
- *Surprise!* For kids, tuck a puzzle, cartoon, or note inside, to say you care.

September 12 Make Room for Mushrooms

Shiitake, crimini, portabella, enoki, oyster, morels, wood ears, or white—whether tossed in a salad, arranged on a pizza or polenta, added to a stir-fry, or stirred into pasta, stew, or soup, mushrooms add earthy flavors.

Nutritionally, mushrooms are low in calories, cholesterol-free, and essentially fat- and sodium-free. They provide many *B vitamins; potassium,* which promotes heart health; *selenium,* an antioxidant that may be heart-healthy; and *copper,* a partner to iron in building red blood cells. Mushrooms may supply cancer-protective phytonutrients.

Tip: For best flavor, refrigerate them in paper bags or covered with paper towels; enjoy them at their peak freshness.

During National Mushroom Month, prepare a dish with specialty mushrooms for distinctive flavors.

Portopasta

6 to 8 ounces portabella mushrooms
2 tablespoons olive oil
½ cup chopped onion
½ cup chopped sweet red pepper
1 teaspoon minced garlic

2 cups prepared marinara sauce
8 ounces pasta, cooked according
   to package directions
Salt and pepper to taste

Slice portabellas. In a large skillet, heat oil. Add portabellas, onion, red pepper, and garlic; cook and stir until mushrooms are tender, 5 to 6 minutes. Stir in prepared sauce; heat until hot, about 3 minutes. Add pasta; toss until well combined. Season with salt and pepper to taste. Makes 4 (1½-cup) portions.
Source: Mushroom Council

September 13   Cook Savvy—Seven Ways to Fast Forward

Back in the hectic swing of things with summer nearly over? Cook smart—even if you run in ten directions on a 24/7 schedule!
Fast forward healthful eating for your family table.

- *Stock up.* Buy quick-to-fix ingredients: canned and frozen fruit, vegetables, beans; pasta and rice; yogurt and cheese; canned soup; pasta sauces; partly prepared ingredients (salad kits, stir-fry–ready vegetables, oven-ready marinated packaged meat).
- *Keep simple.* No-cook dishes—sandwiches, tuna or bean salads—can be as healthful as time-consuming ones.
- *Double or triple batch.* Cook enough for today and later: meat sauce for spaghetti tonight and for potato toppers later.
- *Serve do-it-yourself meals.* Set out ingredients for others to assemble—pizza, sandwiches, tacos, fajitas, chef salads.
- *Crock it.* Use a slow cooker to braise food slowly while you do other things.
- *Cook when time allows.* Freeze stews, casseroles, and meat sauces for later use.
- *Involve your family.* Even table setting, pouring milk, or tossing a salad is a time saver and a chance to nurture kids' kitchen skills!

September 14 Insider Trading

Did summer leisure relax your resolve to eat smart? If so, now's a great time to get back on track, with an eat-smart strategy to try: food trade-offs.

Trading off means thinking about all your food choices for a day, then substituting. For a food with more fat, sugar, salt, or calories, trade in a similar food with less. Or limit more indulgent foods; spend the savings elsewhere. The idea is to moderate and balance, not eliminate.

Try these food trade-offs, or come up with your own:

- *For calories:* Eat a half (not a whole) brownie at lunch. Spend some calorie savings on a small fruit smoothie later. *Strategy: Limit portion size.*
- *For fat:* Eat a salsa-topped baked potato instead of fries. Spend some fat savings on a cheese-and-cracker snack later. *Strategy: Substitute another food later.*
- *For fat:* Choose grilled chicken breast instead of breaded chicken nuggets. *Strategy: Substitute a healthier version.*
- *For sugar:* Drink one soda today, not two. Spend some sugar savings on an oatmeal cookie. *Strategy: Limit how often.*

September 15 Nourish Your Mind

This semester, why not bone up on nutrition with a reliable health guide to shelve between your favorite cookbook and your family medical book? Although covers may be eye-catching, you can't always judge a book by its cover alone. Look deeper.

- *Author's credentials.* Is the author a well-respected professional, such as an RD (registered dietitian) or a DTR (dietetic technician, registered), with a degree in nutrition, medicine, or related specialty from an accredited college or university?
- *Reviewers' credentials.* Is there a list of peer reviewers with their credentials?
- *Published to inform.* Is the book a serious work, not for product promotion only?

- *Credible sources cited.* Has the author used research or advice from government agencies, respected universities, peer-reviewed scientific journals, and credible professional and health organizations?

To find a nutrition book with scientifically sound, consumer-focused advice:

- *Check the American Dietetic Association's Web site* (www.eatright. org) for recommended titles and as a gateway to other reliable titles.
- *Call a local nutrition expert:* a registered dietitian or other qualified nutritionist who may work at a college, hospital, Cooperative Extension office, or public health department. Find the Extension or public health office under Government in your phone book.

September 16   Bowled Over

Ready for two-way convenience in a healthful meal? Go for one-dish dining—one nutrient-rich dish to prepare, one pot to wash!

In both restaurants and supermarkets, "food bowls" and other one-dish prepared meals are attracting time-pressed diners. Yet the cost for fully prepared convenience may be five to ten times more per pound for what's inside. Why not put stove top–casserole convenience in your kitchen?

Bowl over your family with quick, easy, flavorful dinner "bowls."

- *Buy convenience:* presliced vegetables, precut ground lean meat or poultry, herb blends, prepared sauces.
- *Skip the side dish.* Mix your veggies or fruit into one-dish stir-fries, stews, and casseroles.

Lemony Beef and Barley with Sugar Snap Peas

1 pound lean ground beef	½ cup quick-cooking barley
½ pound mushrooms, sliced	½ teaspoon salt
1 medium onion, chopped	¼ teaspoon pepper
1 large carrot, thinly sliced	1 8-ounce package frozen sugar
1 clove garlic, crushed	snap peas, defrosted
1 13⅔- to 14½-ounce can ready-to-serve beef broth	¼ cup chopped fresh parsley
	1 teaspoon grated lemon peel

In large nonstick skillet, cook and stir ground beef, mushrooms, onion, carrot, and garlic over medium heat 8 to 10 minutes or until beef is no longer pink, breaking up beef into ¾-inch crumbles. Pour off drippings. Stir in broth, barley, salt, and pepper. Bring to a boil; reduce heat to medium-low. Cover tightly and simmer 10 minutes. Add peas; continue cooking 2 to 5 minutes or until barley is tender. Stir in parsley and lemon peel. Makes 4 (1¾-cup) servings.

Source: Cattlemen's Beef Board and National Cattlemen's Beef Association

September 17   ✍   Play Grounds

Are you a coffee drinker? If you're among the majority of Americans who are, how does coffee fit into your fitness plan?

The weight of scientific evidence indicates that moderate coffee and caffeine intake (200 to 300 milligrams daily) poses no health problems. And there's no scientific link to cancer, fibrocystic breast disease, heart disease, ulcers, infertility, birth defects, or osteoporosis. What about high blood pressure (hypertension)? The National Heart, Lung and Blood Institute notes that caffeine may cause a temporary rise in blood pressure. But unless you're caffeine sensitive, you don't need to limit caffeine to prevent hypertension or control blood pressure. Under current scientific study is whether there are any phytonutrient benefits from substances in coffee.

Of course, if caffeine gives you jitters or insomnia, go easy. (*Note:* Eight ounces of brewed coffee have on average 85 milligrams caffeine; an ounce of espresso, about 40 milligrams.)

Add flavor and nutrition to your coffee cup.

- *Enjoy south-of-the-border coffee,* where "regular" coffee is mostly milk. Fill a fourth of your mug with coffee, top with warm milk.
- *Order a 12-ounce café latte, mocha, or cappuccino* for 250 or more milligrams of calcium.
- *Re-create your java.* Turn coffee that gets cold in your mug into iced latte—just add milk and ice.
- *Chill out with a coffee smoothie.* Blend ½ banana, ¼ cup espresso, ¼ cup milk, 1 scoop coffee or vanilla ice cream, 1 cup ice, and a pinch of nutmeg or cinnamon.

September 18   🍴 Eat Thin

Need to trim a few pounds, or avoid gaining any more? Try these tricks of the savvy weight trade:

- *Serve on a salad plate.* Less looks like more.
- *Start low.* Eat salads, vegetables, and other lower-calorie foods first. Smaller portions of higher-calorie foods follow.
- *Pick foods you chew.* Eat fruit, instead of juice. Fiber is filling.
- *Sup on soup.* Add extra veggies to clear or noncreamy soups to make them heartier.
- *Switch from whole to 1% low-fat milk.* Save 50 calories daily per 8-ounce cup.
- *Cut down on caloric drinks*—soda, lemonade, sugary tea, fruit drinks. One less 20-ounce soda saves about 270 calories daily, or 98,550 calories per year!
- *Skip mayo.* Flavor with mustard.
- *Limit alcoholic drinks.* Have no more than one a day, or weekends only. Alcohol is *not* calorie-free.
- *See your food.* Eat from a plate, not the package. Then you know how much you really eat.
- *Eat only when you're hungry.*
- *Eat until you're nearly full.* Savor how good you feel to be satisfied, not stuffed.

September 19   🍴 A Real Fish Story

Don't let that big one get away!

Omega-3s in fish—and some plant-based foods—help promote heart health, which is one reason why the American Heart Association (AHA) advises eating fish, particularly fatty fish, at least twice weekly. Albacore tuna, anchovies, herring, lake trout, mackerel, salmon, and swordfish are among those with the most. Tofu, other soy foods, canola, walnuts, flaxseeds, and their oils have omega-3s, too, in lesser amounts.

Benefits? Omega-3s may help lower blood triglycerides (unhealthy blood fat), reduce plaque buildup in arteries, reduce blood clots (risky for heart attacks and strokes), lower blood pressure, and lower the chance of fatal irregular heartbeat.

With such promising benefits from omega-3s, the AHA advises fish oil under a doctor's supervision for some people. Before using it, ask your physician if it's right for you. Since too much fish oil may cause bleeding, caution is essential.

Eating a variety of fish helps reduce possible adverse effects of any water pollutants. Children and pregnant and nursing women should exercise caution with fatty fish, which may contain higher mercury levels.

To "lure" two meals of fatty fish into your weekly menu:

- *Start your day with smoked salmon (lox)*—on a bagel, in an omelet.
- *Make "tuna" salad with canned mackerel.*
- *Order anchovies on your pizza.*

Swordfish Piccata

½ teaspoon black pepper
1 pound swordfish, ½-in. thick cutlets (or steaks)
1 tablespoon finely chopped parsley

2 tablespoons lemon juice
2 teaspoons capers
Lemon slices

Pepper swordfish, and place on a broiling pan. Broil fish for 1½ minutes on each side or until flesh turns opaque. Remove swordfish from broiling pan, and place on a heated serving platter. Sprinkle with parsley, lemon juice, and capers. Garnish with lemon slices. Makes 4 servings.
Source: California Seafood Council

September 20   Fig-ure This Out

What flower looks like a fruit and was enjoyed as training food and trophy by ancient Olympian athletes? Figs!

Figs are a terrific source of both *insoluble* and *soluble fiber,* aiding digestion and helping to lower cholesterol levels. What's more, they supply some *potassium, iron,* and *calcium*—more than other fruits.

And figs contain *polyphenol antioxidants,* with potentially health-promoting benefits. Harvesttime is late summer to early fall—peak season for fresh figs.

Experiment with figs—fresh or dried—in your meals.

- *Sweeten vegetables.* Add sliced figs to cooked sweet potatoes, green beans, roasted onions, or squash.
- *Make salads elegant.* Slice figs; toss with Caesar, Waldorf, slaw, or garden salad.
- *Make batter better.* Mix finely chopped figs into buttermilk pancake or muffin batter.
- *Flavor cooked grains.* Stir chopped figs into rice, couscous, or barley during cooking; for more flavor, add sautéed onions and herbs, too.

September 21 Looks Like Water, Sold Like Water, But . . .

Remember when tap water was the only water? Now marketers tout health benefits of another so-called option: waters enhanced with vitamins, minerals, and herbs. Are they any better for you? Despite claims, probably not.

First, the calories: Added sugars flavor many enhanced waters, and the calories add up. Second, the add-ins: Do you really need their vitamins or minerals? Not if you're already getting enough from food and a daily supplement. And herbal add-ins are full of unknowns: unknown effectiveness; unknown interactions with food, medicine, supplements; unknown safe dosages.

Enjoy the fresh, pure flavor of icy-cold plain water—as refreshing as it gets! If you like flavor:

- *Flavor any water, still or sparkling.* Add a slice of citrus fruit, or a fresh sprig of herb, perhaps mint. Or add your own fruit-juice ice cubes.
- *Buy calorie-free flavored seltzer.*

September 22 Passport to Health—Eating Italian Style

Bon appetito! Italian pasta, risotto, and polenta not only deliver complex carbs. They're also perfect partners for a colorful array of veggies, fiber-rich legumes, and small portions of meat, poultry, and fish. The fat? Mostly heart-healthier monounsaturated olive oil.

For an Italian-style flavor today:

- *Add fagioli (white beans)* to minestrone soup or pasta sauce.
- *Prepare arborio (short-grain) rice* with sautéed vegetables, cooked shrimp, or grated cheese.
- *Try this easy Italian-inspired snack!*

Easy Bruschetta

1 cup shredded mozzarella cheese	salt and pepper, to taste
2 cloves garlic, finely chopped	1 large ready-to-eat pizza crust (or similar bread)*
1 cup diced tomato	
8 fresh basil leaves, sliced thin in strips, or 2 teaspoons dried basil	

Preheat oven to 375°F. Toss together cheese, garlic, tomato, basil, salt, and pepper. Spread mixture on top of pizza crust. Place on baking sheet, and bake for 8 to 10 minutes or until cheese is melted. Cut into slices and serve immediately. Makes 4 to 6 servings.

Source: American Dairy Association

*For more fiber, use whole-wheat crust, bread, or pita.

September 23 Kids—In Motion?

Did you know that children spend on average 17 hours a week watching television? That leisure computer time often replaces active play? That inactive children more likely become inactive adults? That today many overweight kids already show early signs of cardiovascular disease, diabetes, and high blood pressure?

Despite the popular interest in fitness, today's youths are less fit than the last generation. Studies that track kids' fitness note less strength and less endurance when running. Childhood obesity is up.

Most kids don't engage in regular physical activity that promotes long-term health and a healthy weight. Many schools no longer require daily physical education, and few promote lifelong active living.

Now during back-to-school time, advocate for active lifestyles for kids.

- *Speak out for daily physical activity at school*—at parents' meetings, in school newsletters, and with administrators and your school board.
- *Support active after-school activities*—in Scouting, Boys and Girls Clubs, sports clubs, and other community programs.
- *Encourage kids to be active at home*—by limiting television and leisure computer time and by planning active family time.

September 24   Go the Extra Smile

Laughter not only diffuses negative emotions and stress. It may also change your body's chemistry—so you really may laugh your troubles away.

The reasons are not yet understood. However, laughter may reduce stress hormones—epinephrine and cortisol—which tend to impair the protective lining of blood vessels. Without that protection, the chance of cholesterol buildup and heart disease is higher. A few good laughs releases muscle tension and endorphins. And they may also boost immunity with more production of infection-fighting antibodies, help protect against cancer, and may increase tolerance to pain. And with a smile, you look younger and feel better, too.

Find something to prompt laughter in your life today.

- *Keep humor in view.* At your workplace, hang a cartoon, photo, or quote that makes you giggle.
- *Rent a funny movie; watch your favorite sitcom.*
- *Learn to laugh at youself.* You'll give others permission to laugh *with* you.

September 25   "All You Can Eat"

Sounds like a deal! Or is it? An average salad bar plate can easily add up to 1,000 calories—more if you pile on dressing, cheese, bacon bits, nuts, and more.

If self-control is your challenge, pass on all-you-can-eat buffets and salad bars.

To help with self-control, try this:

- *Survey first.* Check the buffet options from end-to-end before you pick up those tongs.
- *Start with a salad trip only.* That takes the edge off your hunger. Next trip, go easy on non-salad items, especially creamy soups, bread spreads, desserts.
- *Make a one-plate promise.* That doesn't mean cramming food in every space!
- *Use only small plates.* Forget the dinner-size plate, especially if you tend to overfill it. Go easy with the dressing ladle.
- *Take a little at a time.* You *can* go back if you're still hungry. Besides, when your plate's not mounded, you can truly enjoy distinctive flavors from each food.

September 26   Autumn's Do List

You can burn as many calories (about 150) with 30 to 40 minutes of raking or gardening as you can with a 5-mile, 30-minute bike ride. Point is, you don't need to leave home to benefit from moderate activity.

With summer over, gather your supplies, and set aside time this weekend for physically active household projects.

- *Do household fix-ups yourself.* Painting, wallpapering, building, and landscaping may keep you in nearly constant motion.
- *Refinish furniture.* A little elbow grease may turn a worn-out garage sale find into a household treasure.
- *Clean your garage, attic, or basement.* Hauling, sweeping, boxing up, and rearranging uses plenty of muscle and motion.

September 27   Rating Your Risk

A new health report says "doubles your risk," "proves that . . . ," "significant finding." What's your *real* risk?

That depends. If your risk was one in a million, then "double the risk" is still very low, at one in 500,000. But if your risk was one in 100, then "double" truly is a big increase! With terms like "proves," take caution. A small handful of studies rarely proves anything. And "significant" may or may not mean "important." Instead "statistically significant" means a mathematical association.

Not sure how to interpret what you hear on today's health news?

- *Listen to actual numbers.* Real incidence, not just relative incidence, is important to know if you're at risk.
- *Check with a credible expert.* To find a local nutrition professional, contact your local Extension office or hospital or click onto www.eatright.org.

September 28   Squash That Idea

Ready to "season" your family meal with autumn flavor and color? Winter squash adds both. Their hard yet edible skin and more intense flavors distinguish acorn, butternut, pumpkin, buttercup, calabaza, golden nugget, and turban squash from tender-skinned, mild-flavored summer squash.

The inside scoop makes a great nutrition story. The deep-yellow to deep-orange flesh offers more nutrients, *fiber,* and other phytonutrients than summer squash, notably more *beta carotene* and *lutein* (two antioxidants), more *soluble* and *insoluble fiber* (helps control cholesterol levels and promote elimination), and more *thiamin* and *vitamin B$_6$, potassium,* and *iron.* It's also a low-fat source of another antioxidant: *vitamin E.*

Enjoy winter squash . . .

- *Peeled and cut up cooked in pasta sauces, soups, and stews*
- *Mashed and seasoned with cinnamon and nutmeg*
- *Cooked and tossed with other cooked veggies.*

Spicy Apple-Filled Squash

1 acorn squash (about 1 pound)	⅛ teaspoon ground cinnamon
1 apple, peeled, cored, and sliced	⅛ teaspoon ground nutmeg
2 teaspoons melted margarine	Dash of ground cloves
2 teaspoons packed brown sugar	

Heat oven to 350°F. Grease a baking dish. Halve squash and remove seeds; bake 35 minutes. Keep oven on. Cut squash halves in two; turn cut sides up. In small bowl, combine apple, margarine, brown sugar, cinnamon, nutmeg, and cloves, and mix well. Fill squash pieces with apple mixture. Cover with foil or lid; bake 30 minutes or until apples are tender. Makes 4 servings.
Source: Washington State Apple Commission

September 29 Meat—Shop "Skinny"

Think you need to take meat off your menu to eat lean? Not so. Just keep portions sensible, and buy the leanest meat you can. Beef's a great source of *protein, iron, zinc,* and *B vitamins.* And 3 ounces of cooked beef round (size of a deck of cards) has 4 fat grams and 2 grams of saturated fat (comparable to 3 ounces of skinless dark and light meat chicken).

To put the leanest meat in your cart this week:

- *Know clues to lean cuts:* "round" and "loin" for beef, "loin" and "leg" for pork and lamb.
- *Shop "select" grades.* "Select" for beef (and "good" for veal and lamb) has less fat between the muscle; "prime" has the most. Except for fat, protein and other nutrient content comes out the same.
- *Buy well-trimmed meat.* Just ⅛ inch or less in the outside fat layer.
- *Buy leaner ground beef.* Ground round is leanest, then ground sirloin, then chuck, then regular ground beef.
- *Ask the butcher.* Ask for a leaner cut or a closer trim.

September 30 Hands Clean?

Did you know that the simple habit of frequent handwashing during food prep could cut the incidence of food-borne illness in half?

What's the risk? Though invisible to the naked eye, "unfriendly" bacteria on your hands easily pass from raw meat or poultry to other surfaces in the kitchen: utensil handles, appliance knobs, counter-tops, and dishrags. Unwashed hands and contaminated equipment transfer bacteria to raw fruits and vegetables, breads, and other uncooked foods.

Make handwashing a habit during National Food Safety Education Month—and beyond.

- *Wash often* in warm, soapy water before preparing foods and especially after handling raw meat, poultry, and seafood.
- *Wash when you switch kitchen tasks* between handling raw meat and cutting vegetables.
- *Wash after other things you do*—for example, after taking out garbage, after sneezing, and after petting your dog.
- *Wash well for 20 seconds*—the front and back of your hands, up to your wrists, between fingers, and under fingernails.
- *Wash with warm water and any soap.* There's no difference between antibacterial and ordinary soap in reducing the spread of food-borne illness.
- *Dry with care* using disposable paper towels or clean towels.

October 1   Love Pasta?

If you're a pasta fan, you'll enjoy these factoids this National Pasta Month: Americans eat pasta for dinner forty times yearly. About 600 pasta shapes exist worldwide. The Chinese ate pasta 5,000 years ago; Italians, more than 1,500 years before Marco Polo's time.

Now more facts and tips: To cook pasta, use 1 quart of boiling water per 4 ounces of dry pasta. Stir occasionally as pasta comes to a boil. Salt cooking water *only* if you want to. Skip rinsing after cooking, unless you're not saucing it right away or using it for a salad.

Remember, 4 cups of cooked pasta equals 8 ounces of uncooked long pasta shapes (a 1½-inch-diameter bunch); 1 cup cooked pasta is two Bread Group servings.

As you shop for pasta:

- *Enjoy the fun shapes and flavors:* bowties, spirals, twists, wheels, and tomato- or spinach-flavored pastas. (The flavoring gives hardly any nutrition boost.)
- *Match pasta with sauces:* angel hair with light, thin sauces; fettuccine with heavier sauces; penne or irregular shapes with chunkier sauces.
- *Try wheat-free pasta for something different:* made with barley, bean threads, buckwheat, oats, rice, or potato starch. If you have celiac disease (gluten intolerance) or a wheat allergy, read the ingredient list to be sure it's wheat- and gluten-free.
- *Need to watch egg yolks?* Skip egg noodles if you have an egg allergy; read the ingredient list to check.

October 2   Charge It

How do you recharge when a midafternoon slump hits? With coffee, a power drink, or a candy bar? Other better-for-you options may be more effective.

An afternoon slump may be part of your body rhythm, even if you get enough rest, eat smart, stay active, and manage stress. According to new research, high-carbohydrate meals may increase seratonin among some people and so contribute to drowsiness.

To keep your energy up midday:

- *Eat lunch even when you're under pressure.* Erratic eating can be an energy robber.
- *Power up.* Include lunch foods that stick with you longer: a chef's salad with meat, poultry, cheese, nuts, or tofu.
- *Snack smart if you're hungry.* Keep nutrient-rich snacks handy in your work area: fruit, juice, whole-wheat pretzels, yogurt, trail mix.
- *Skip martini lunches.* Alcoholic drinks may make you drowsy.
- *Get up.* Maybe you need to move, not eat. Walk to a colleague's desk to rev up your metabolism.

- *Change your pace.* Switch tasks to challenge your mind with something different. If your energy level is usually higher in the morning, plan more demanding work then. If your job allows, try a 15-minute nap.
- *Dump stress.* It zaps energy. (See April 15.)

October 3 Veggies for Dessert

With creativity you can fit veggies anywhere into any meal—even dessert!

Carrots, pumpkin, and sweet potatoes, rich in beta carotene, make great dessert ingredients; enjoy them in Southern-style pudding. Corn and zucchini appear in sweet breads; tofu, in cheesecake and frozen desserts; rhubarb in pie; even cucumber in a refreshing sorbet!

For vegetables in your dessert menu:

- *Blend a pumpkin smoothie.* Whirl canned pumpkin, fat-free milk, frozen vanilla yogurt, a dash of pumpkin pie spice or cinnamon in a blender.
- *Use carrot juice* as the liquid in baked goods. It won't taste like carrots!

Chocolate Zucchini Muffins

1½ cups all-purpose flour
¼ cup unsweetened cocoa powder
1 teaspoon salt
1 teaspoon baking soda
½ teaspoon baking powder
¼ cup ground flaxseed
½ cup margarine

¼ cup vegetable oil
1½ cups sugar
2 eggs
½ cup buttermilk
2 cups finely grated unpeeled zucchini

Preheat oven to 350°F. In a bowl, combine flour, cocoa, salt, baking soda, baking powder, and ground flaxseed. In a separate bowl, cream margarine, oil, and sugar. Add eggs and buttermilk. Add flour mixture, stirring until just mixed. Add zucchini and mix. Fill paper baking cups half to two-thirds full. Bake 18 to 20 minutes or until wooden pick inserted in center comes out clean. Remove and cool on rack. Makes 24 muffins.
Source: Flax Council of Canada

October 4 🍎 Garlic and Onions—Breath-taking Advice

Crisp, juicy onions; firm, smooth garlic cloves; long, fibrous leeks: great for flavor, bad for your breath, likely good for your heart.

What makes the onion family (onions, garlic, leeks, chives, scallions) so flavorful and so healthful is their *allyl sulfides*, one type of phytonutrient. According to today's research, these aromatic compounds may help to lower LDL- (bad) cholesterol, control blood pressure, prevent blood clotting (in blood vessels), act as antioxidants to reduce cancer risk, and perhaps promote immunity.

Tip: for the health benefits, enjoy onions and garlic, not just garlic powder, onion salt, or garlic oil or pills. For garlic, you likely need at least one clove daily to make a difference.

If these pungent foods offend your nose or tastebuds:

- *Rub odor away.* Wipe your hands with salt or lemon juice after handling.
- *Hold your tears.* Refrigerate onions before cutting them.
- *Lessen the flavor.* Pour boiling, then cold, water over raw onions. Or cook to mellow.
- *Freshen your breath.* Eat the parsley garnish. Or sip ginger or mint tea afterward.

October 5 ⚕ Breast Cancer—Be Aware

Did you know that eventually every woman is at risk for breast cancer, just by getting older? A family history of breast cancer increases the risk. In any case, if you're a female, consider nutrition-focused strategies to lower your risk.

- *Keep a healthy weight.* Gaining extra weight during adulthood, especially during pregnancy, seems to increase the risk.
- *Stay physically active.* It helps prevent weight gain. Exercise may moderate estrogen levels, too. Estrogen doesn't cause cancer, but it may stimulate cell growth.
- *Eat five to nine servings of fruits and vegetables daily.* Their antioxidant properties may be cancer-protective.

- *Trim fat.* Limit saturated fat and keep trans fats as low as possible without compromising good nutrition. That may lower colon and breast cancer risks.
- *Limit alcoholic drinks.* For women, no more than one drink (wine, beer, or distilled spirits) daily is best. Two or more increases the risk slightly. Those with high risk should avoid alcohol altogether.

What about soy? The research link isn't clear. Isoflavones in soy foods seem to block estrogen from promoting tumors. For women at high risk for estrogen-dependent breast cancer, just *moderate* amounts of soy foods are advised. But isoflavone supplements aren't. Large doses may be harmful.

During this National Breast Cancer Awareness Month:

- *Women:* Take one action to reduce your breast cancer risk today. Perhaps schedule a mammogram.
- *Men:* Offer encouragement to a woman you care about. (*Note:* Men are at risk, too.)

October 6   Which Bread Is "Whole"?

Brown or the multigrain bread is not necessarily whole-grain. The rich brown color may come from caramel coloring, not from whole-grain flour.

For the record, if it's labeled "whole wheat," bread must be made from 100 percent whole-wheat flour. However, "wheat bread" may contain some refined white flour. Proportions vary. Oat, corn, and rye flours are whole-grain, too.

To find bread with more fiber, check two spots on the label:

1. *Nutrition Facts* for fiber content. A slice of whole-wheat bread has about 2 grams of fiber unless fiber-fortified; a slice of white, about 0.6 grams of fiber. (Daily fiber advice is: men, 30 to 38 grams; women, 21 to 25 grams, depending on age. Kids' levels are figured as age plus five—that's 18 grams for someone age 13.)

2. *Ingredient list* for whole-wheat or other whole-grain flours. They should be first or second on the list.

If you pack an autumn picnic next weekend, make sandwiches with:

- *Rye bagel,* layered with lean turkey ham, Cheddar cheese, shredded cabbage, and mustard
- *Crusty oatmeal bread,* filled with salmon salad and baby spinach leaves
- *Whole-wheat hot dog buns,* wrapped around grilled lean sausages, topped with salsa

October 7   Pizzazz in Your Pizza

Is pizza good for you? Sure, especially if you eat just what you need (likely a couple of slices). One slice (⅛ of a 12-inch pizza) may supply about 185 calories and 5 to 7 fat grams; half of the same pizza, about 750 calories and 20 to 30 fat grams. Remember, cheese has bone-building calcium; tomato sauce has several antioxidants, including beta carotene, vitamin C, and lycopene.

October is National Pizza Month. If oven-ready pizza's on tonight's menu, give it pizzazz (and a few more nutrients). Top pizza with flavorful, nutritious extras to help you eat five to nine servings of fruits and veggies daily.

- *Load on the greens:* chopped broccoli, shredded spinach, snow peas, sliced zucchini.
- *Pepper with flavor:* red, yellow, and green peppers. Fore more taste excitement, try Anaheim peppers, or even hotter jalapeños!
- *"Veg it up" even more:* shredded carrots, sliced shiitake mushrooms, asparagus spears, kidney beans or any beans, even leftover vegetables.

October 8   Scaled Down?

Dining alone? Rather than simply "forage" when you're hungry, bored, or lonely, redesign your meal approach to eat smart, boost your appetite, and avoid emotional overeating or undereating. You're worth it!

Make solo meals worth the work.

- *Plan small, but smart.* Shop ahead for easy-to-fix, healthful meals. Perhaps buy meal or salad kits, partly prepared for you.
- *Buy single-portioned food:* small amounts of produce, portioned meat or fish, canned soup or fruit "singles."
- *Minimize the effort.* Cook once; eat twice. Enjoy half a broiled chicken tonight; use the rest on a Caesar salad tomorrow.
- *Make meal dates.* Invite a friend or a family member to eat with you, or take a meal to them. Enjoy potluck meals or brown bag breakfasts or lunches together.
- *Turn eating into a special event*—away from the countertop. Turn on music. Use your dishes, not just the microwave container.

October 9   Hurry Up and Wait

Standing and waiting, sitting and waiting—so much unproductive time in sedentary activity. Why not use all that waiting time effectively?

Multitask by moving rather than just waiting.

- *Skip the drive-thru.* Park instead, and walk inside to order food, cash a check, or pick up a prescription.
- *Climb the stairs* when it's just a few flights.
- *Walk on the moving sidewalk.* You'll arrive even faster.
- *Sweep the floor* while your microwave lunch heats up.
- *Stretch or bend* while you wait for your computer to boot up or download.
- *Take a walk* while you wait for a car repair or, if you're early, for a personal appointment.
- *If you must wait, stand.* You burn more calories standing than sitting down!

October 10   Cook Savvy—Lean Ways to Cook

Trying to cook with less fat? Try these techniques:

- *Braise or stew* over low heat in liquid with a tight-fitting lid.

- *Broil or grill* with direct heat, often over hot coals.
- *Microwave* with no fat added.
- *Roast* uncovered in the oven, with dry heat.
- *Simmer or poach* slowly in liquid, just below boiling.
- *Steam* over, but not in, boiling water.

For the record, frying, especially deep-fat frying, is high-fat cooking! If you're in a hurry, stir-fry at high heat in just a little fat, stirring often. Cook in a low-fat way tonight.

Hurry Curry Stir-Fry

1 tablespoon vegetable oil	1 teaspoon grated fresh ginger
¾ pound beef sirloin steak, cut into 1-inch-thick slices	1 teaspoon curry powder
1 medium onion, chopped	¾ teaspoon salt
1 clove garlic, minced	2 medium baking apples, coarsely chopped
3 cups cooked brown rice*	¼ cup apple cider or apple juice
½ cup slivered almonds, toasted	

Heat oil in large skillet over medium-high heat until hot. Add beef, onion, and garlic; cook, stirring constantly, 5 to 7 minutes or until beef is no longer pink. Add rice, almonds, ginger, curry powder, and salt. Cook and stir 3 minutes, or until flavors are well blended. Just before serving, stir in apples and apple cider. Makes 6 servings.

Source: USA Rice Federation

*For convenience, cook brown rice ahead; refrigerate up to 7 days.

October 11   Got Kids?

Help your child get a lunchtime *A* for nourishment to learn.

For a packed lunch, have kids help plan and pack their lunch (in a cool-looking carry container). They'll more likely eat it. Pack variety (and a frozen chill-pack to keep perishable foods safe): a sandwich, left-over chicken legs, even cold pizza; fruit (kiwi, starfruit, and grapes are fun); cut-up raw veggies; celery with peanut butter; whole-wheat crackers or an oatmeal cookie; milk money. Tuck in a "You're great!" note.

For meals served at school, check what's served at your child's school. By regulation, schools that participate in the National School Lunch Program must offer a variety, with fruit, vegetables, and milk. Schools may offer other options, too, including fast food, à la carte items, and vending machine foods. Buying a school lunch may cost less than home-made, and may de-stress your morning "rush hour."

Kids celebrate National School Lunch Week at school in October—join in!

- *Talk together about the school menu.* Help your child practice making choices; include milk. Talk about new foods.
- *Volunteer in the cafeteria.* Schools need help with cafeteria events, new food tastings, and daily mealtimes.
- *Find out about the school's nutrition education.* Reinforce at home what your child learns at school.

October 12   An Apple a Day

There's truth in the time-honored adage that an apple a day keeps the doctor away.

Enjoy a crunchy, medium-size apple *with its peel on,* and get the benefits of about 4 grams of dietary fiber in just 80 calories. That's about 15 percent of the amount advised daily for adults. An apple's mostly *soluble fiber* may help lower blood cholesterol levels by binding to fatty substances and promoting their excretion. Its *insoluble fiber* helps waste move through your intestinal tract faster.

Other sweet benefits? Apples, especially their peels, are loaded with quercetin. A powerful antioxidant, *quercetin* may reduce the growth and spread of cancer cells, and help promote heart health by protecting your blood vessels from fatty deposits. What's more, *tannins* in apple juice may help keep your gums healthy.

Another "a-peeling" fact: aroma and flavor mostly come from fragrance cells in the peel. *Vitamin C* is just underneath.

Enjoy apples to celebrate National Apple Month in October.

- *Toss in some apple crunch.* Add chopped sweet red or tart green apple to a garden or chicken salad or tuna salad sandwich.
- *Tuck in an apple.* Pack a whole apple, dried apple slices, or canned apple juice in your briefcase or backpack.
- *Spread chunky applesauce* on your morning French toast, pancakes, or waffles, instead of syrup.

October 13   Pick It Up, Slow It Down

Interval workouts aren't just for serious athletes. If your physical activity routine gets boring or if the challenge disappears, pick it up and slow it down in repeated intervals.

Anyone can get more health benefits and burn more calories—and have more fun—by alternating light, moderate, and more strenuous activity. Just remember: warm up slowly, cool down slowly at the end. Skip the urge to push too hard, too often.

To make any activity more demanding, move longer, move more, or push harder.

- *Do it your way.* If you're a beginner, slow walk, *then* walk, *then* slow walk. Work up at *your* pace.
- *Turn up your current routine.* If you circle the track or the neighborhood, step faster every two to three minutes, then slow down to less demanding action. An up-and-down course makes an interval workout on a bicycle easier.
- *Program your fitness equipment for interval training* if the equipment provides this computerized feature. Try the uphill feature.

October 14   Think Vegetarian

Roasted vegetables with sesame seeds, grilled portabella and pepper panini, cilantro rice and beans with ancho chilies. You don't need to be an everyday vegetarian to enjoy appealing vegetable dishes. But if you are, you may enjoy the benefits of plant-based eating—if you choose foods carefully.

The chance of heart disease, high blood pressure, type 2 diabetes, some cancers, even obesity tends to be lower among vegetarians. Typically they eat less saturated fat and cholesterol, and more complex carbohydrates, fiber, folate, and phytonutrients. Protein sources differ, but they can be just as adequate in protein as meat.

But beware, vegetarian eating *can* be high-fat or high-calorie, too. Soy burgers, soy hot dogs, and other vegetarian dishes can have high-fat ingredients. Other challenges: A vegetarian diet may come up short in iron and zinc, vitamin B$_{12}$ (found only in meat, pountry, fish, and dairy foods), and perhaps calcium and vitamin D when dairy foods aren't consumed.

Enjoy easy vegetarian meals during National Vegetarian Awareness Month.

- *Grill meaty portabella mushrooms* to make great mushroom burgers.
- *Transform spaghetti* with canned kidney, cannellini, or soybeans in place of meatballs.
- *Load your pizza* with frozen or canned mixed veggies and beans or tempeh.
- *Toss nuts* into vegetable salads and stir-fries.

October 15   Health E-Advice

Need instant nutrition information? E-nutrition advice is just a few mouse clicks away. How do you know what's trustworthy when search engines list legitimate and less reliable sites side-by-side?

Media savvy doesn't apply just to magazines, newspapers, TV, radio, and books. Exercise the same healthy skepticism you would with any resource. (See August 20, September 15, November 29.) To judge nutrition cyber-advice:

- *Identify the Web site sponsor* and the sites it links to. Suffixes offer a clue to the source: *.org* (associations), *.edu* (educational institutions), *.gov* (government), *.com* (commercial). To appear credible, any Web site may hyperlink to expert sites. Commercial (.com) sites, with a marketing focusing, may—or may not—offer credible information to educate consumers.
- *Check for updates.* Reliable sources are updated frequently. (Less reliable sources may be, too.)
- *Look for a rating:* Tufts Nutrition Navigator—www.navigator. tufts.edu—offers trustworthy ratings.
- *Ask for an expert critique.* A registered dietitian (RD) or dietetic technician, registered (DTR) can give you a science-based perspective.

- *Determine the Web site's main objective.* Is it education or primarily advertising?

To find science-based online advice quickly, use a gateway, linked to many responsible organizations and Web sites.

- *U.S. government:* www.healthfinder.gov and www.nutrition.gov
- *American Dietetic Association:* www.eatright.org

October 16   🛒 $$ Smart

In the United States, about $36 per week per person is spent on groceries. Get the most nutrition for your dollars with nutrient-dense foods. Consider: two melons cost about the same as two 64-ounce bottles of soda; a large bag of chips, about the same as a bag of apples. Exercise supermarket savvy.

- *Buy it your way.* If you don't need a whole package of meat, seafood, or produce, ask the butcher or clerk to repackage just the amount you need.
- *Clip coupons.* And check the Internet for money-saving promos. Buy *only* if you need the item, and if it's really a better price.
- *Pay attention to the unit price displayed on the shelf.* Buy a bigger size if it keeps well.
- *Buy the quality you need.* You don't need gourmet olive oil for everyday food prep.
- *Consider the cost of convenience.* Lettuce may cost three times more if it's cut up and prewashed. Worth it? That's your call.

October 17   🍎 On the Wild Side

Ready to go wild with your meals? Enjoy the nutty flavor and good nutrition of wild rice. Combine 1 cup raw wild rice with 3 (or 4) cups water, bring to a boil, then simmer, covered, for 30 to 45 minutes; you're done! Cooked wild rice can be refrigerated for about one week.

Wild rice isn't rice, but instead an edible seed with more than twice the *protein* of brown or white rice—more *iron* and *fiber,* too.

Get wild today.

- *Add cooked wild rice* to soups, leftover vegetables, or ground meat for burgers.
- *Enjoy it* as you would cooked oatmeal for breakfast.

Northwest Asparagus Wild Rice Salad

1 cup uncooked wild rice	*Dressing*:*
3 cups thinly sliced fresh or frozen asparagus	¼ cup white wine vinegar
4 ounces cut-up smoked salmon	1 tablespoon olive oil
1 cup cranberries	1 tablespoon Dijon-style mustard
1 cup sliced red bell pepper	½ teaspoon salt

Cook wild rice to package directions. Rinse in cold water. Combine asparagus, salmon, cranberries, red bell pepper, and cooked rice. Mix well. Combine dressing ingredients. Toss dressing with salad. Makes 4 to 6 servings.

Source: Washington Asparagus Commission

*Bottled dressing, such as Cranberry-Ginger Vinaigrette, may be substituted.

October 18 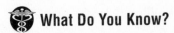 What Do You Know?

Do you buy into food myths? Here are three true-or-false questions to test your thinking.

1. Spicy foods cause ulcers.
2. Sugar causes diabetes.
3. Fasting cleans the body of toxins.

All three statements are *false.* Surprised?

Ulcers are caused by the *Heliobactor pylori* bacteria. Chilies and other spices promote mucus formation that helps protect the stomach lining.

People with diabetes can't use sugar or other carbohydrates in a normal way. The causes of diabetes are complex and linked to overweight, genetics, illness, inactivity, and just getting older.

Your liver and kidneys "detox" your body constantly. Fasting doesn't do that; to the contrary, ketones build up when carbohydrates aren't available for energy.

To help you sort nutrition facts from myths:

- *Seek advice from qualified experts:* among reliable sources, a registered dietitian (RD) or a dietetic technician, registered (DTR).
- *Ready to learn more?* Click on to this Web site for daily healthful eating tips: www.eatright.org.

October 19   Keep Compu-Fit

Do you feel computer fatigue after a workday? For the tiny muscles that control your eyes as you view the screen and the big muscles that support your back as you sit, your body needs regular breaks from extended computer work. You need good lighting (no glare, good contrast), a chair that allows for good posture, and a computer positioned for comfort, too.

Take short, frequent breaks. ('Net surfing isn't a break!)

- *For your eyes:* Blink frequently. Close your eyes occasionally for a few moments. Every 15 minutes or so, look away from the computer screen at a distant object.
- *For your hands and arms:* Take a minute to use different muscles. Stretch. Stand up and take a few deep breaths.
- *For your whole body:* Get up from your workstation and move for at least 5 minutes every 60 minutes. During your midday break, take a brisk walk—15 minutes or more to promote your overall fitness.

October 20   Cereal for Breakfast?

What cereal is right for you? With more than a hundred varieties, you've got choices!

Check for fiber. Pick higher-fiber cereals—with perhaps whole wheat, bran, or oats as the first ingredient. Check serving size, too. Breakfast cereals may contain a range from 0.5 to 10 fiber grams per ounce. Daily fiber goal? Age 50 or under: 25 grams for women, 38 grams for men, and slightly less (21 grams for women, 30 grams for men) if you're older.

Analyze claims. Be sensible about highly fortified cereals (with calcium, antioxidants, B vitamins, iron, and/or zinc). One hundred percent of everything isn't necessary, especially if you take a multivitamin/ mineral supplement, too. Herbal add-ins? Promised benefits are iffy.

Look for trans fat. Most cereals are low in fat. Unhealthy trans fat (partly hydrogenated fat) may appear in granola, among others.

With any breakfast cereal:

- *Drink your cereal milk*—for *all* the calcium benefits in the bowl.
- *Sweeten with fruit*—for vitamin C, beta carotene, fiber, and other nutrient and phytonutrient benefits, too.
- *Top with yogurt*—if you like cold cereal crunch. Besides its calcium, yogurt with active live cultures has probiotic benefits. (See July 19.)
- *Sprinkle on nuts*—for more fiber and phytonutrient benefits.

October 21 ☤ Keeping Regular

Though not brought up in "polite" conversation, regular elimination signals your good health—now *and* later. Regular differs from person to person. For most folks, one or two soft, bulky stools daily is normal.

It's not surprising that health risks rise when elimination isn't normal. The chances for hemorrhoids and diverticulosis go up as hard stools put pressure on the colon and the rectum. Colon cancer risk may rise, too, since food waste (with potentially harmful substances) that moves too slowly through your intestines has more time to contact intestinal walls.

To keep regular, take stock of your everyday habits.

- *Drink enough.* Dehydration contributes to hard, dry stools.
- *Listen to your body's signals.* Delaying can lead to constipation.
- *Eat plenty of fiber-rich foods.* Fiber helps soften and bulk up waste so it passes through your intestines with ease and normal frequency. (See August 3.)
- *Stay physically active.* Active living helps keep muscle tone throughout your whole body—your intestinal tract, too.
- *If these habits still don't work? Talk to your doctor.*

October 22 Your Pork-folio

"Lean-ing" toward health? If you eat meat, how about a pork dinner tonight? A 3-ounce cooked lean pork loin chop has about 170 calories and 65 grams of cholesterol. Compare that to 150 calories and 70 grams of cholesterol in 3 ounces of cooked, skinless chicken breast.

To keep pork dishes lean and flavorful: Buy lean pork cuts—tenderloin, loin, sirloin, or rib cuts—and trim away any fat you see before cooking. Marinate for more flavor. Control portions—a 3-ounce cooked portion is the size of a deck of cards. Cook the low-fat way—broil, grill, roast, or stir-fry in just a little fat—to a safe internal temperature of 160°F (that's medium, not well done).

Here's an easy soup made with pork to enjoy during National Pork Month:

Spicy Tortilla Soup

½ pound lean ground pork
½ cup chopped onion
1 28-ounce can crushed tomatoes
1 15-ounce can chicken broth
1 8-ounce jar medium-hot salsa
1 teaspoon ground cumin

1 teaspoon chili powder
½ teaspoon salt
½ teaspoon garlic powder
½ teaspoon ground black pepper
4 corn tortillas, cut into thin strips

Brown pork and onions over medium-high heat in large nonstick saucepan, stirring occasionally. Add remaining ingredients except tortilla strips. Cover and simmer 20 minutes. Stir tortilla strips into soup, and simmer for 5 to 10 minutes more, until tortilla strips are softened. Makes 6 servings.
Source: National Pork Board

October 23 ☤ Got the Creeps?

Is your weight creeping up? Caloric needs drop with age—about 2 percent a decade—so your eating should slow down, too.

Before you blame your slowing metabolism on hormone changes alone, give credit to loss of muscle cell mass, too. After age 20, most adults lose about one-half pound of muscle per year. And a sedentary lifestyle may leave you with less energy-burning muscle cells.

Good news about strength training: you *can* rebuild muscle mass at any age and so speed your metabolism. Other benefits: lower chance of injury, and everyday tasks get easier to do.

Start building strength today.

- *Talk to your physician before starting strength training.* Learn what's safe for you.
- *Find a certified fitness professional.* To find the right-for-you strength-training program, ask your physician for a reference.
- *Build strength training into daily tasks.* Carry groceries, do yard work, walk up and down stairs.

October 24   Eat Ethnic

Enjoy taste adventures? They're a good health strategy, too. More and more consumers are caught up in the culinary trend. A willingness to try new grain products, fruits, and vegetables (including ethnic flavors) gives you more ways to fit forty or so different nutrients, as well as thousands of health-promoting phytonutrients, into your personal food style.

Celebrate United Nations Day by reaching beyond your basics to taste ethnic foods.

- *Shop the ethnic food aisle in your supermarket.* Or find an ethnic food store, often a great place for tips on preparing unfamiliar ingredients.
- *Invite a foreign guest to dinner, perhaps an exchange student.* Cook his or her family recipes together.
- *Buy an ethnic cookbook.* Experiment with its recipes.
- *Plan a culinary vacation.* In fact, any trip, long or short, can introduce you to new foods and flavors if you're ready for a taste adventure.
- *Sign up for an ethnic cooking class.* Or watch one on TV.
- *Find a unique ethnic restaurant.* Eat there instead of your everyday favorite once in a while.

October 25 Packed Your Sneakers?

Do you stick to your fitness routine when you travel? If so, great! Still, you know it isn't always easy. The next time you take a trip—whether for business or pleasure—take steps to keep your fitness plan on track.

Some travel fitness tips:

- *For your trip planning,* book a hotel with a fitness area. Belong to a health club? See if the club offers benefits elsewhere.
- *As you pack,* tuck in athletic shoes and comfortable clothes, and perhaps a bathing suit or a jump rope. Bring a headset and tapes to enjoy while you walk or jog.
- *On your way,* walk the airport concourse; skip people movers. Take regular walk-and-stretch breaks if you drive.
- *After you arrive,* get a local walking map—then walk to business meetings, tourist sites, and restaurants. Start or end your day with a power walk or a jog. Work out in your hotel room with a televised fitness program.

October 26 Seed-y Side of Health

Seeds of hope, seeds of wisdom, seeds of change—seeds carry potential! So it's no surprise that plant seeds are also a concentrated nutrient source.

You probably eat more seeds than you think. There are seeds *for flavoring:* caraway, cardamom, celery, coriander, cumin, mustard, and sesame seeds; seeds *as vegetables:* beans and peas. Some seeds are a *rice alternate:* wild rice (see October 17). And seeds can be a *fat substitute:* flaxseed (see August 10).

Consider the health-promoting benefits of flaxseed, and pumpkin, sesame, and sunflower seeds. Although high in fat, it's mostly the heart-healthy *unsaturated kind.* Seeds are also good *fiber* and *protein* sources, especially for strict vegetarians. And they supply varying amounts of *iron, magnesium, potassium, zinc,* and other *minerals.*

Add "seeds of change" to your meals and snacks.

- *Toss*—in a spinach or mixed green salad.
- *Sprinkle*—over hot or ready-to-eat cereal.
- *Mix*—into meat, turkey, or tuna loaf or patties, and casseroles.
- *Stir-fry*—with vegetables.

October 27 Passport to Health—Eating Spanish Style

With health-focused interest in Mediterranean eating, Spanish-style cooking is drawing attention. Its flavor profile features olive oil, a mostly monounsaturated fat, and garlic with its possible heart-healthy benefits, too. Many dishes call for seafood, also heart-healthy. And meals feature ingredients with complex carbs—rice, potatoes, and bread. Among other signature ingredients: green and red peppers, tomatoes, ground almonds (in soups, sauces, desserts), cured ham, and chorizo sausage.

Prepare a Spain-inspired dish today.

Spanish Omelet

1 tablespoon butter*
½ cup frozen cubed potatoes, thawed
2 tablespoons chopped onion
¼ cup diced sweet red pepper
1 clove garlic, minced
3 eggs
3 tablespoons water

2 tablespoons minced parsley
¼ teaspoon salt
Dash pepper
2 tablespoons sliced pitted green olives
2 tablespoons shredded Cheddar cheese

In 10-inch nonstick skillet over medium heat, heat butter. Cook potatoes, onion, pepper, and garlic until tender, about 8 minutes. In small bowl, beat eggs, water, parsley, salt, and pepper until well blended; pour over vegetables. With spatula, carefully push cooked portions at edges toward center so uncooked portions can reach hot pan surface, tilting pan and moving cooked portion as necessary. When top is thickened and no visible liquid egg remains, sprinkle with olives and cheese. With spatula, fold omelet in half. Invert onto plate with a quick flip of the wrist or slide from pan onto plate. Cut in half. Makes 2 servings.

Source: American Egg Board

*Or olive oil.

October 28 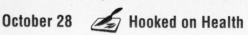 Hooked on Health

Hooked on seafood at least twice a week? That's heart-healthy advice from nutrition experts. Compared with many other protein foods, most seafood (finfish and shellfish) has less calories and fat, and certainly less saturated fat. And polyunsaturated omega-3 fatty acids in fatty fish (dark-fleshed albacore tuna, mackerel, and salmon) may promote heart health.

Note: Children and pregnant and nursing women need caution with king mackerel, swordfish, shark, and tilefish, which may contain higher mercury levels.

October is National Seafood Month. Explore easy ways to enjoy fish and shellfish.

- *Switch places.* Substitute fish for meat or poultry in salads, soups, casseroles, pasta dishes, and stir-fries.
- *Reinvent your burger.* Try canned salmon, tuna, crabmeat, or mackerel in place of ground beef in burgers and meatloaf.
- *Wrap some fish tacos.* Flavor grilled, broiled, or canned fish with lime juice and garlic; tuck into soft warm tacos with cilantro, chopped pepper, and onion.
- *Cook creatively.* Poach fish in wine and herb-seasoned broth. Marinate chunks of meatier fish (swordfish, halibut, fresh tuna) on skewers with vegetable chunks and then grill. Barbecue fish with your favorite sauce.
- *Create crispy baked (not fried) fish.* Dip fillets in a mustard-milk mixture, roll them in ground pecans, and bake in a nonstick baking dish.

October 29 Picking a Multi

Need a supplement, or not? A low-dose multi (to avoid nutrient overload) may be good insurance, although the best nutrition guideline is always "food first."

A multi *won't* provide energy, since vitamins and minerals have no calories; fiber, since it's not a nutrient; phytonutrients from plant-based foods that help promote health and protect against disease; nutrients not listed on the label.

A multi *will* provide low doses of key vitamins and minerals to fill your nutrition gaps. See January 6.

If you buy a multi:

- *Stick to 100% Daily Value.* That's enough from one dose. Your food choices provide plenty of nutrition already.
- *Men and postmenopausal women:* Buy a supplement with low or no iron. Iron from supplements meant for premenopausal women can build to dangerous levels.
- *Consider natural vitamin E.* Look for "d-alpha-tocopherol" on the label. It's better absorbed than synthetic.
- *Check the calcium level.* It's not enough to substitute for calcium-rich foods.
- *Buy the generic brand.*
- *Avoid doubling up* if you take a single-nutrient supplement, too.
- *At home, store supplements safely,* securely closed, out of kids' reach. (Adult iron supplements are the main cause of poisoning deaths among children in the United States.)

October 30    Just Add You

Little effort, plenty of nutrition. Why not turn a quick side dish, like a boxed rice or grain mix, into an easy main dish? Simply fortify it with generous amounts of vegetables and a high-protein ingredient.

A few tips: (1) use half the seasoning packet, which is likely high in sodium; (2) switch from butter or margarine to vegetable or olive oil for less saturated fat; (3) add vegetables toward the end of cooking for more color, crisp texture, and vitamin retention; and (4) cook in low-sodium broth instead of water for more flavor.

Start with a whole-grain mix (barley, brown rice, whole-wheat couscous,) for more fiber. Mix in what you like.

- *Canned fish* (packed in water, not oil) *or poultry:* chicken, crab-meat, salmon, shrimp, tuna

- *Canned beans:* any kind. Rinse for less sodium, or buy those with less salt or sodium.
- *Dried fruit:* cranberries, currants, raisins, or chopped apples, apricots, plums (prunes)
- *Herbs (fresh or dried):* basil, chili powder, chives, cilantro, dill, parsley, oregano
- *Nuts or seeds:* almonds, peanuts, pecans, pine nuts, pistachios, walnuts; sunflower or sesame seeds
- *Tofu:* firm or extra firm, perhaps flavored
- *Vegetables:* canned, fresh, or frozen. Buy them precut from the salad bar or produce department.
- *Cheese (added just before serving), if you'd like:* perhaps reduced-fat types or a little Parmesan, feta, sharp Cheddar, or other strong-flavored cheese

October 31   Treat, or Trick?

Ghosts and goblins, carved pumpkins, masks, candy—how will you celebrate this ghoulish day? Enjoy a modest, not oversized, portion of candy. Skip mindless noshing on candy that's around after Halloween.

Will trick-or-treat candy affect kids' behavior? Probably not. Any overactive behavior more likely comes from excited anticipation and Halloween parties, costumes, and other fun. No scientific evidence confirms a link between sugary snacks and hyperactivity. Nonetheless, help your child go easy on sugary snacks and add a reminder: Brush teeth after any snack.

For other "be-witching" ways to enjoy the day:

- *Offer noncandy treats:* boxed raisins, packets of nuts or pretzels, apples.
- *Teach self-discipline with snacks.* Help kids ration their Halloween booty—just one small portion a day. It's fun to stretch the festivity!
- *Brew up a quick, active Halloween get-together-for kids or adults.* Bob for apples. Act out charades or "scary stories." Serve apple juice (hot or cold), popcorn, pumpkin or oatmeal cookies, or make-your-own pizza (decorated with a scary face) with veggies.

November 1   Cranberries—Not Just for Holidays

Do cranberries conjure up thoughts of the holidays? Whether you drink cranberry juice, blend canned cranberries in smoothies, add cranberries to poultry or pork stuffing, or enjoy cranberries in salsas, salads, or side dishes, cranberries help keep you healthy any time of year. They're loaded with *vitamin C* and other *antioxidants.*

Their crimson color comes from a *flavonoid* that may help lower your LDL- (bad) cholesterol, help prevent blood clots that cause heart attacks and stroke—and so protect you from heart disease. Their other plant substances may protect you from some cancers, gum disease, and stomach ulcers.

Another better-known benefit: Substances in cranberries help prevent bacteria in the urinary tract from causing bladder infections.

Mix cranberries—fresh, frozen, or dried—into batters and doughs.

Cranberry Bread

½ cup butter	1 teaspoon baking soda
1 cup sugar	¼ teaspoon salt
1 tablespoon grated orange peel	¾ cup buttermilk
1 teaspoon vanilla	2 cups fresh or frozen cranberries,
3 large eggs, beaten	chopped
2½ cups flour	¾ cup pecans, chopped

Preheat oven to 350°F. Spray bottom only of a 9-by-5-inch loaf pan with cooking spray. Beat butter, sugar, orange peel, and vanilla in a large bowl until light and fluffy. Add eggs, mixing well. Combine flour, baking soda, and salt; add to creamed mixture alternately with buttermilk, beating at low speed just until blended. Fold cranberries and nuts into batter. Turn into prepared pan, spreading evenly. Bake until wooden pick inserted in center comes out clean, about 50 to 60 minutes. Cool slightly in pan. Remove from pan and cool completely on wire rack. Makes 1 loaf.

Source: Cape Cod Cranberry Growers' Association

November 2   Elect Nutrition

Cast your ballot at the polls yet? Which of the following will you elect to drop into your supermarket cart? Vote true or false as part of your personal campaign for smart eating.

☐ Sugar-free cookies are calorie-free.

☐ Baked chips have a lot fewer calories than regular chips.

☐ A frozen vegetarian entrée is always better for you.

☐ Low-fat foods offer better nutrition.

☐ Fruit drinks count as fruit servings.

All the statements are false! Sugar-free cookies don't have sucrose, but get their calories from other carbs, fats, and proteins. The difference in chips usually isn't that much: 150 calories per ounce of regular chips compared to 120 calories for baked chips. "Vegetarian" means no meat, poultry, or fish; a vegetarian entrée may have cheese or high-fat sauces that bring up the calories and fat. Low-fat foods don't necessarily offer better nutrition, and the calories (from more carbohydrates) may equal that of full-fat versions. Fruit drinks are basically flavored, sweetened water; although they might be fortified with vitamin C, they don't have all the nutrients that juice does.

Be informed today as you "vote with your dollars" for good nutrition.

- *Be skeptical about your own "healthy food" assumptions.*
- *Read the fine print.* Compare products, using the Nutrition Facts on the labels, before you buy.

November 3   ✎ Sandwich in Variety

Tired of packing the same old sandwich for work? Today is Sandwich Day, honoring the seventeenth-century British Earl of Sandwich, who, as legend goes, demanded one-handed meals during his card gambling spree. A perfect day for creative sandwich making!

Make over your lunch sandwiches for more flavor and nutrition.

- *Pick a great wrapper:* whole-wheat, tomato, or spinach tortillas; multigrain, rye, or whole-wheat bread; focaccia; whole-wheat pita; bagel; naan.
- *Switch your filling:* grilled tempeh; lean smoked turkey, pancetta, corned beef; salmon salad; Edam, Gruyère, Havarti, fontina; soy cheese; sliced tofu.

- *Layer in color:* green, red, and yellow pepper slices; shredded carrots; cucumber and tomato slices; spinach leaves; red onion; avocado.
- *Flavor with creativity:* chutney; mustard; horseradish; hummus; light pesto; balsamic vinaigrette; wasabi; chopped cilantro, basil, or other herbs.
- *Sprinkle in crunch:* chopped almonds or walnuts, dried fruit, sunflower seeds.

November 4 Cross-Train, Less Pain

Suffer ongoing soreness? Losing interest in your physical activity routine? Want to take your fitness level up a notch? Then cross-train.

Why cross-train? *By adding variety to your workout,* you work different muscles, which helps make your whole body stronger, more flexible, and perhaps more fit. You won't strain the same muscles, bones, and joints, reducing your chances of injury. Best of all, cross-training is more interesting and more fun, so you're more likely stay with it.

Consider cross-training this week:

- *Alternate from day to day.* Walk one day. Bicycle, swim, or dance the next.
- *Add something different to your regular routine.* If you walk, add 5 minutes of jumping rope or stair stepping.
- *Switch activities within your workout.* At a gym, you might do 10 minutes on a treadmill, 5 minutes on a stationary bike, and 5 minutes on a rowing machine. At home, you might walk briskly for 10 minutes, do calisthenics for 5 minutes, then flexibility exercises for 5 minutes.

November 5 Pre-Diabetes—At Risk?

Do you know your fasting blood sugar level? With the rise in diabetes, health experts advise you to pay attention. Why? Because pre-diabetes usually develops to diabetes. Even during this early stage, long-term cardiovascular damage may occur without notice.

Usually symptom-free, pre-diabetes is blood sugar level that's higher than normal (110 to 125 mg/dL), but not high enough for diagnosis as diabetes (over 125 mg/dL). (A normal blood sugar level is 70 to 110 mg/dL.)

Are you at risk? The odds go up if any of these factors describe you: over age 45; a close family member with diabetes; African American, Hispanic, Asian American, Pacific Islander, or Native American descent; overweight or obese; physically inactive; low HDL- cholesterol or high triglycerides; or gestational diabetes, or delivering a baby weighing 9 pounds or more.

This National Diabetes Month:

- *Have your blood sugar level checked.* Get treatment before pre-diabetes becomes diabetes.
- *Reduce your risk.* Fit in 60 minutes of moderate activity daily if you can. Eat smart to achieve or maintain your healthy weight.

November 6   I Get By with a Little Help from My Friends

Going it alone is hard for most of us, no matter what life's challenges! According to research studies, a "support team" is key to helping many people reach and maintain their health goals. If you need to manage diabetes, a food allergy, high blood pressure, or some other health problem, support often makes a strict eating regimen easier to follow.

If you don't have a support team:

- *Create one! Get a lunch partner.* Eat smart together. Split large restaurant portions. Or take turns bringing healthful bag lunches to share.
- *Join a support group.* Besides the psychological support, it's a great place to swap realistic nutrition strategies.
- *Enlist family support.* Family members not only encourage you; they can also help stock the kitchen with foods you need to eat smart. Return the favor.

November 7 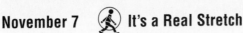 It's a Real Stretch

Know the "tight" feeling that often goes with stress? Or the uncomfortable stiffness that comes from sitting in one place too long? Then stretch! Exercise physiologists say stretching:

- *Promotes relaxation*
- *Improves blood flow*
- *Helps your body feel more flexible,* which reduces muscle injury
- *Keeps your muscles from tightening up after exercise*

For benefits without injury, stretch when your muscles are warmed up. Stretch gently and slowly; it's okay to feel tightness, not pain. Hold for several seconds (no bouncing).

Stretch anywhere, anytime. Start with these easy stretches at work, as you watch TV, or while you talk on the phone:

- *Stand and stretch,* reach for the ceiling.
- *Roll your shoulders* forward and backward, then lift (shrug) and bring them down.
- *Sit and lean forward,* bringing your chest and head between your legs. Put your hands on your feet.
- *Or find a stretching class* that includes breathing and relaxation, perhaps yoga, Pilates, Tai Chi, or "gentle stretching" geared for older adults.

November 8   Fit Veggies In

Vegetables are a nutritional gold mine! So you may buy them. But by week's end is your "garden-fresh" produce wilted in the fridge? Is it perhaps because you're not sure how to prepare them, you don't have the time, or simply that veggies are not in your meal routine?

Here are a few ideas for fitting veggies into your meals while they're still fresh—and at their nutritional and flavor peak.

- *Go for more time-saving.* Buy prewashed, cut-up vegetables.
- *Add extra veggies to convenience soup and stew.* Mix veggies into chicken-noodle soup; add canned beans or bell pepper to corn chowder.

- *Get creative with bagged baby spinach:* on sandwiches, heated in soups, wilted in pasta or risotto, cooked as a pizza topper.
- *Tuck tomatoes and other chopped vegetables:* in burritos, tacos, pita pockets, wraps.
- *Layer atop veggies:* grilled meat, fish, and chicken on a bed of diced carrots, squash, or peppers.
- *Toss salad with any vegetables:* beets, jicama, zucchini, beans, leftovers.
- *Load your pizza:* Fortify store-bought frozen pizza with extra veggies.

November 9 Passport to Health—Eating Middle Eastern Style

Another flavor adventure? If you've eaten at a Middle Eastern restaurant, you may recognize these flavors: carbohydrate-rich rice, bulgur, or couscous in stuffings, salads, side dishes; calcium-rich yogurt in soups and drinks; goat's-milk cheese on salads; fresh and dried fruits, fiber-rich legumes, and nuts as common ingredients; mint, coriander, and cinnamon to season it all.

Experience Middle Eastern–inspired flavors this week.

- *Enjoy store-bought hummus* or make your own. Purée canned chickpeas (garbanzos), garlic, tahini or sesame seeds, lemon juice, and pepper. Sprinkle with parsley; spread on a whole-wheat pita. Check online for a recipe.
- *Mix a yogurt sauce* with plain yogurt, garlic, fresh mint, and ground pepper to spoon over cucumbers or cooked vegetables.

Lamb Kebabs with Mint

1 cup plain low-fat yogurt
½ cup fresh mint, chopped
2 tablespoons Dijon mustard
3 cloves garlic, minced
2 tablespoons lemon juice
Salt (optional) and pepper to taste
14-ounces boneless leg of lamb, fat removed, cubed

4 small zucchini, cut in 1-inch chunks
4 plum tomatoes, halved
2 cups cooked couscous or brown rice

Mix yogurt, mint, mustard, garlic, lemon juice, salt, and pepper in a medium-sized bowl. (Reserve some marinade for basting later.) Add lamb pieces and refrigerate overnight. Preheat broiler or barbecue grill. Thread lamb with zucchini and tomatoes onto skewers. Broil or grill. Cook until desired doneness, turning and basting with marinade, approximately 7 to 10 minutes. Serve over couscous or rice. Makes 4 servings.
Source: Produce for Better Health Foundation

November 10 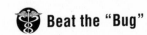 Beat the "Bug"

The flu season is at your doorstep. How can you protect yourself? The best defense is a year-round offense: Eat smart, stay active, get enough rest, reduce stress.

Which nutrients enhance immunity? Several may play key roles: beta carotene in deep-yellow fruits and veggies and dark-green leafy greens; vitamin B_6 in whole grains, legumes, chicken, and pork; vitamin C in citrus fruit, berries, melon, tomatoes, and broccoli; vitamin E in wheat germ and nuts; protein in dairy foods, meat, poultry, fish, and legumes; selenium in meat and seafood; zinc in beef and seafood. Friendly bacteria in yogurt with live cultures also help build immunity.

Herbals? Use caution. Taken longer than several weeks, some herbals (including echinacea and panax ginseng) *may* lower immunity.

Focus on at least one immune-enhancing strategy today.

- *Eat smart: five to nine fruits and vegetable servings daily.* Make one high in vitamin C. Vitamin E in nuts and seeds also helps build immunity.
- *Take a multivitamin/mineral supplement*—if you need a "nutrition safety net." Be aware: High doses don't superimmunize.
- *Schedule a flu shot*—if your doctor recommends it.
- *Get enough sleep*—on average, eight hours daily.
- *Find ways to reduce stress*—perhaps through physical activity, meditation, or simply "time out" from stressors.
- *Move more*—another reason for 60 minutes of active living daily.

November 11   Ancient Secrets

Corn, peanuts, peppers, pineapples, potatoes, tomatoes, wild rice—where would world cuisine be today without the nutrient-rich native foods that first nourished Native Americans?

To commemorate Native American Heritage Month, buy quinoa (keen-WAH), a grainlike food that sustained the Incas five thousand years ago. It's noted for its high *protein* content, as well as its *riboflavin, vitamin E, iron, magnesium, potassium, zinc,* and *fiber.*

To cook whole-grain quinoa: Rinse it first to remove saponins that give a bitter taste, then cook it like rice. Simmer 1 cup quinoa in 2 cups water, covered, for about 15 minutes, until the water is absorbed. The grain will turn transparent. (Look for quinoa sold as flour, pasta, and flakes, too.)

Recipe call for rice or barley? Use quinoa instead.

- *In pilaf:* For a nutty flavor, brown it in a dry skillet for 5 minutes, then cook it.
- *In salads:* Toss quinoa with cooked shrimp, celery, walnuts, dried cranberries, and low-fat salad dressing.
- *In soups:* Thicken turkey soup with quinoa.

November 12   Class Act

Got a great kitchen, but don't use all its features? Cooking classes may be for you!

If you're new to the kitchen, consider a class in culinary basics, or perhaps knife skills. Already a "foodie"? Learn ethnic or regional cuisine. And if you need to manage a health issue, check your local hospital for community classes, perhaps on cooking for heart health, diabetes, or gluten intolerance.

Get your culinary juices flowing.

- *Sign up for "couples cook."* Married or single, cooking classes make great date nights.
- *Give a culinary gift certificate*—to a family member, maybe a child or a teen.

- *Learn at home.* Watch cooking demos on TV or with video clips online.
- *Plan a culinary vacation.* Cooking schools and culinary festivals are popping up everywhere. What a great way to learn the ethnic flavor of your destination—and bring it back to your kitchen!
- *Throw a cooking class party at home.* Invite a food-savvy friend to teach, or chip in for a local instructor.
- *Take your party to a cooking school.* Arrange for a private group class.

November 13 Herbals Safe?

Herbals are not necessarily safe, even though they're natural. Although many herbal supplements probably are safe, their use is still full of unknowns. (See August 22.) *Some* are known to have hazardous, even deadly, side effects. It's best to avoid these.

Herbal Supplement	Possible Side Effects
chaparral	liver damage
comfrey	liver damage, possible carcinogen
ephedra/ma huang	dizziness, changes in blood pressure, rapid heartbeat, heart attack, stroke, nerve damage, others, even death
germander	liver damage, possible death
kombucha	possible death
lobelia	breathing problems, rapid heartbeat, low blood pressure, coma, even death
magnolia/stephania	kidney damage
willow bark	Reye's syndrome in children, allergic reaction
wormwood	nerve damage, arm/leg numbness, delirium, paralysis
yohimbe	anxiety, paralysis, gastrointestinal problems, psychosis

If you take herbal supplements, do this today:

- *Check the label.* If any contain the hazardous ingredients listed above, stop taking them.
- *Keep on checking.* Other herbals are toxic, too. Check with your physician.
- *Remember this red flag:* If you're on medications or undergoing any type of surgery, consult your doctor and pharmacist before you take *any* herbals!

November 14 Video Tonight?

Busy schedule mean there's no time for the gym? No fitness center nearby or cost too much? Prefer working out on your own? You still can fit in workouts. Borrow, buy, or rent an exercise video; work out on your schedule, in the privacy of your home.

Stores stock dozens of exercise videotapes. Picking the right one for you is like finding the right workout class. Here are four things to look for. It should:

1. Feature a certified instructor who inspires you, not just a celebrity.
2. Include adequate warm-up and cool-down activities.
3. Match your abilities so you don't get frustrated.
4. Provide alternative moves that may be easier.

Before you buy any workout video, read its package to see if it might require any special equipment, such as steps, stretch rope, weights.

Now—ready, set, start!

- *Make space.* Move small furniture and "stuff" so you have enough room to move.
- *Watch the videotape first.* Once you've seen the motions and their patterns, rewind the tape and work out.
- *Do it at your pace.* Modify the moves if they're too intense for you. Gradually pick up your pace as you use the videotape again and again.

November 15 🖊 Cook Savvy—Sweet Story

Have a sweet tooth? Try satisfying it with more nutrient-rich fruit and fewer foods with added sugars.

Sweeten your day as you cook.

- *Enhance fruit's sweetness with heat.* Stuff a cored apple with cinnamon, dried berries, and nuts; bake at 350°F until slightly softened. Poach pears in fruit juice; top with toasted nuts.
- *Choose unsweetened cereal.* Sweeten with fruit.
- *Top pancakes, French toast, and waffles with fruit purée.* Swirl fresh, frozen, or canned fruit in a blender; thin with juice. Use fruit purée as a glaze for meat, poultry, or fish, too.
- *Toss fruit in garden salads:* dried cranberries, blueberries, or cherries, or cut-up fresh fruit.
- *Add a sweet perception.* Some ingredients bring out sweetness: vanilla, peppermint, other extracts. So do "sweet" spices and herbs: cardamom, cinnamon, coriander, ginger, lavender, mace, nutmeg, mint.
- *Opt for canned fruit in natural juices.* Look for canned fruit, flavored with "sweet" spices, too.
- *Cook with quick-frozen fruit, no added sugars.*
- *Buy unflavored yogurt.* Sweeten with chopped fruit, berries, fruit purée.
- *Add sweet garnishes:* berries or diced fruit on sweet potatoes, pumpkin soup, broiled seafood.

November 16 🥂 Party or Not—Drink Responsibly

Do you enjoy a celebration drink during the holiday season? Remember the year-round guideline for moderation: no more than one drink daily for women, two for men. The key to moderation is knowing alcohol equivalency. One standard drink (12 ounces beer, or 5 ounces wine, or 1½ ounces 80-proof distilled spirits) has about 14 grams of alcohol.

If you drink alcoholic beverages—or someone you socialize with does—these tips promote responsible drinking:

- *Eat first.* That slows alcohol absorption.
- *Set your limit from the start.* Stick to it.
- *Make the first drink nonalcoholic*—perhaps a "virgin" cocktail (nonalcoholic mixers) to quench your thirst.
- *Ask for ice.* It ups the volume and dilutes the drink.
- *Set down your drink.* You'll talk more and sip less.
- *Drink water, still or sparkling, when you're thirsty.* Alcoholic beverages are dehydrating.
- *Alternate.* Have a nonalcoholic drink after one with alcohol. Give your body the hour it needs to detoxify a standard-size drink.
- *Never drink if it puts you or others at risk!*

November 17 Going Bananas

Simple to enjoy, great to pack and carry, healthful to eat—bananas are among America's most popular fruits.

On average, American consumers eat about 84 bananas yearly! What's under the peel? Among other substances, *potassium,* which helps reduce the risk of high blood pressure and stroke; *vitamin C,* not only an immunity builder, but an antioxidant with health-protecting benefits, too; *fiber,* linked to reduced risk of cancer and heart disease; and more digestible *carbohydrates* than any other fruit has.

Grab a banana today—or bake a batch of banana bran muffins.

Banana Bran Muffins

¾ cup whole-bran cereal
¼ cup milk
3 ripe bananas
1 egg
¼ cup light molasses

2 tablespoons vegetable oil
1 teaspoon baking soda
¼ teaspoon salt
¾ cup raisins

Preheat oven to 375°F. Soften bran cereal in milk. Slice bananas into blender; purée. Combine bananas, egg, molasses, and oil; mix until blended. Combine flour, baking soda, and salt. Stir flour mixture and moistened bran mixture into banana mixture until dry ingredients are just moistened. Fold in raisins. Spoon into well-greased muffin pan (⅓-cup size). Bake 25 to 30 minutes. Makes 12 muffins.

Source: International Banana Association

November 18   Flying High

Traveling home for the holidays? Give thought to airport and airline food and drink. In-flight food service may be only a small bag of dry snacks and a beverage, even if you fly over mealtime.

Pack these thoughts as you pack your bags:

- *Tuck nonperishable snacks into your carry-on bag:* dried fruit, crackers and cheese, raw vegetables, single-serve applesauce or pudding.
- *Look for smart airport food.* Many of today's airports offer flavorful, nutrient-rich, and lower-fat options: wrap sandwiches, packaged salads, smoothies.
- *Let the snack cart roll on by.* If you ate already, you don't need it.
- *Do order from the beverage cart.* Try to have one cup of fluid per hour in flight. Ask for water or buy some to bring along. Dry, recirculating air in a pressurized airline cabin is dehydrating, which in turn promotes jet lag.
- *Go easy on alcoholic drinks, even if they're free.* They promote dehydration and jet lag.

November 19   Turkey Talk

It's nearly Thanksgiving and time to talk turkey—turkey safety, that is! For your meal to bring only compliments, keep turkey flavorful and safe.

- *Keep clean.* Before and after handling raw turkey and its parts, always wash your hands in warm, soapy water. Keep your utensils and work surfaces clean, too.
- *Thaw safely*—in the fridge, on a clean tray, for 24 hours per 5 pounds of whole turkey, or in cold water that's changed every 30 minutes.
- *Stuff with care.* Cooking dressing separately is safest; fill the turkey cavity with onion or apples and herbs instead. If you prefer to stuff, fill the bird loosely *just before roasting:* ¾ cup stuffing per pound of turkey.

- *Cook thoroughly in no less than a 325°F oven. (No partial precooking!)* Use a meat thermometer to check for doneness: 180°F in the thickest part of the thigh muscle, not touching bone, and 165°F for the stuffing.
- *Serve hot, and finish serving within two hours of roasting.* Guests late? Keep cooked turkey hot in a 200°F oven, with the internal temperature at least 140°F.
- *Store leftovers safely.* First remove the stuffing and debone. Refrigerate in shallow containers within two hours of cooking. Eat refrigerated leftover stuffing within two days and turkey within four days.

November 20 How to Be a Thoughtful Host

Hosting a party or overnight guests? Whether or not you know it, some may need to restrict their food choices—for example, people with diabetes or food allergies, vegetarians, or those with religious restrictions. As you plan food for a special occasion, make guests your top priority.

To set a great and flavorful table, keep in mind:

- *When you invite, ask.* Are there foods your guests can't eat? And is timing (perhaps for people with diabetes) an issue?
- *Plan with something for everyone.* Try a vegetable casserole for a vegetarian, or grilled or broiled meat (no heavy sauces) if a guest has diabetes.
- *Invite guests to bring a dish.* That's at least one dish they can enjoy.
- *Ask guests to help with food prep.* Then they can prepare food to match their needs. Serve family style; let guests control their portions.
- *Stick with the meal schedule, if you can.* That's good hosting, and especially important if any guests have diabetes.
- *Skip any bad feelings.* If your "star" dish goes untouched, that's okay. You can still enjoy it, and the leftovers later!

November 21   Buffet Bug Bite?

Entertaining this season? Serve carefully so "buffet bugs" won't bite your guests! That's important for everyone, especially those at higher risk (pregnant women, young children, older guests, or any guest dealing with cancer, HIV or AIDS, or other immunity problems). You might not know who's at risk.

Buffets are perfect breeding grounds for bacteria that cause food-borne illness. What's perishable? Any dish made with meat, poultry, fish, or eggs.

For buffet service, remember these food safety rules:

- *Keep a safe temperature.* Keep hot foods on a warming tray or chafing dish, and cold foods on ice whenever food stays out a while.
- *Replace, not refresh.* Instead of replenishing a dish with fresh food, bring out a new platter or bowl of food.
- *Remember the two-hour rule.* If food sits out longer than two hours, toss; if it soars to 90°F or higher, toss after one hour. (Toss the leftovers, too.)

November 22   The Family Table

Can you get your family together at mealtime at least a few times a week? Research shows that family meals promote healthier eating—more fruits, vegetables, and fiber; less fried food; often fewer calories. And they do far more than put healthful food on the table.

In our haste to get meals prepared, we may forget that mealtime gives time to talk, listen, and build family relationships. And it's a chance for parents to be good role models for healthful eating.

Thanksgiving week and National Family Week—a great time to enjoy at least one meal together as a family! Try to make it routine.

- *Set a regular family mealtime.* Pick a time together.
- *Enjoy more table time, less cooking time.* Make quick, simple meals (even a sandwich, fruit, and milk) to give more table time together.

- *Turn off the TV.* Turn on the phone answering machine. Focus mealtime on family talk.
- *Keep table talk positive.* Everyone gets to talk and to listen. Sitting around a table, not side-by-side at the counter, helps.
- *Keep table time realistic*—not so long that the pleasure goes away.

November 23 Holiday Makeovers

Time for holiday feasting, and you're entitled to a little indulgence. Sure. But just one seasonal feast may add up to a whopping 3,000 calories! Why not make over your holiday meal to bring up the flavor and nutrition, take down the fat and calories, and keep your eat-smart plan on track?

When planning, shopping, cooking—keep these tips in mind:

- *Buy a lean bird, the type that isn't self-basting.* Infused basting ingredients are high in fat.
- *Buy fat-free broth or zesty juice to baste the turkey.* Butter or margarine is not needed.
- *Cook dressing as a side dish.* Add a little broth for moistness. Then it can't absorb turkey fat. Instead, flavor your turkey with fresh herbs (perhaps sage, savory, thyme), gently tucked between the uncooked skin and flesh before roasting.
- *Lighten up the sauce.* Top broccoli with a lemon squeeze rather than Hollandaise.
- *Make it pumpkin.* Usually, pumpkin pie has less fat and sugar than pecan pie, and you get a beta carotene boost, too. Top it with frozen yogurt rather than whipped cream.
- *Wonder about deep-frying your turkey?* Keep the frying temperature high enough—at 350°F—as it cooks, so oil won't seep into the turkey meat. Be cautious with hot oil!

November 24 My Aching Stomach!

Does a sumptuous holiday dinner leave you with an upset stomach or a bloated feeling? (Be careful about blaming the cook.)

Indigestion is certainly caused by digestive diseases. But according to the National Institute of Diabetes and Digestive and Kidney Diseases, indigestion may happen if you:

- Eat too much or too fast
- Eat high-fat foods, such as rich gravy or high-fat desserts
- Eat when you're tired or stressed (Ongoing stress can make indigestion worse.)
- Smoke, especially right before eating
- Drink too many alcoholic beverages
- Exercise too soon on a full stomach (Wait at least an hour.)

For the record, food itself doesn't cause indigestion but may aggravate the problem by stimulating your stomach to make more digestive acids.

If your indigestion is persistent, or if you vomit, sweat, or feel severe abdominal pain, shortness of breath, or pain that travels to your arm, neck, or jaw, see your doctor.

If you're susceptible to indigestion:

- *Heed the best advice:* Avoid foods and situations that seem to cause it. Keep a food diary to find out what they are.
- *Use an antacid*—if it helps.

November 25   Back to Our Roots

Root vegetables, that is, and tubers, too! Besides beets, carrots, potatoes, radishes, and turnips, a lot of nourishing vegetables grow under the ground. Have you ever tried boniato, celeriac, jicama, malanga, salsify, sunchokes, taro, or yuca?

All supply plenty of *complex carbs* and *fiber,* yet virtually no fat. With flavors that range from sweet to earthy, they offer a versatile and economical way to add nourishment and flavor to your plate. Cut and cook them in hearty soups and stews; use them in place of potatoes, perhaps in a potato salad.

Try a new root or tuber veggie. Here's a great way to do that with turkey leftovers:

Turkey Jicama Salad

2 cups diced cooked turkey breast
2 stalks celery, cut up
2 red potatoes, cooked and cut into cubes
⅔ cup diced jicama (or water chestnuts)
3 green onions, cut up

1 tablespoon parsley flakes, or to taste
2 teaspoon dill weed, or to taste
1 cup low-fat plain yogurt
Pepper to taste

Lightly mix the turkey, celery, potatoes, jicama, onions, parsley, and dill. Add the yogurt and mix. Add pepper to taste. Makes 4 servings.

Serve with a roll or on a bed of lettuce.

Source: Produce for Better Health Foundation

November 26 Reinventing Thanksgiving

Nothing tastes better than turkey with all the trimmings! But what to do with leftovers? Reheating is one option. But refrigerate leftover turkey for no more than three or four days, and stuffing for one to two days. And for safety's sake, reheat to 165°F internal temperature. (See April 22 and November 19.)

Another option: Reinvent your Thanksgiving feast a day or two later.

- *Make a hearty harvest stew.* Start with leftover gravy (fat skimmed away before making gravy) as the base. Make it hearty with leftover turkey and veggies. Thicken with mashed potatoes or sweet potatoes. Cook to 165°F for food safety.
- *Stack a turkey-berry wrap.* Wrap sliced turkey, spread with cranberry sauce and shredded greens, in whole-wheat tortillas. Add toasted pecans if you have some.
- *Whirl cranberry smoothies.* Whirl cranberries with frozen yogurt and orange juice.
- *Freeze turkey stock in small amounts.* Later, cook couscous, pasta, rice, or soup with the stock, instead of water.
- *Toss crunchy turkey salad.* Toss cubed turkey with celery, apples, and light mayo with shredded baby spinach.
- *Make stuffing frittata:* stuffing mixed with egg and cooked through, pancake-style.

November 27   Just Jump

Want to feel like a kid again? Get a jump start with a jump rope! You'll get a great cardio workout while you fine-tune your foot-hand coordination. The only expense: a good pair of cross-trainers (shoes with a reinforced toe and good cushioning) and a lightweight jump rope. For the right length rope, step on the rope's center; the handles should stretch to your armpits.

Now for technique. Relax your shoulders. Bring in your elbows. Bend your knees slightly. Twirl the rope smoothly over your head with your wrists. Keep your head up and back straight. Make your jumps low.

Start jumping this week.

- *Begin simply.* Start with a short jumping session; do more as you build your stamina.
- *Jump to music.* Find some upbeat tunes, and jump rope to their beat.
- *Keep twirling.* When you take a break, twirl your rope from side-to-side to keep moving your arms.
- *Learn new jumps.* Get a jump-roping videotape to learn from.
- *Try double Dutch*—perhaps with kids.

November 28   Simple Snackology

Live in a family of snackers? Likely so. On average, 20 to 30 percent of calories consumed by Americans come from snacking—and about 75 percent of us snack!

Snacking itself is okay *when* it fills in the day's nutrition gaps—and *if* you don't overdo on calories, sugars, or fat.

For everybody in your family, smart snacks from your kitchen are very visible, effortless, good-for-you, and flavorful, too.

- *Keep fruit on the counter.* That way, whole fruit's in easy view.
- *Stock smart single-serve, ready-to-go snacks:* small raisin boxes, baby carrots, juice, fruit cups.

- *Wash 'em up.* Get veggies washed, cut-up, and ready to eat from the fridge.
- *Make them visible.* Put fruit and vegetable snacks in see-through containers or plastic bags. That way, your family can spot the smart snacks.
- *Keep smart snacks within kids' easy reach.* Put chips, cookies, and other "sometimes" foods away from impulse eaters.

November 29   Dump the Junk

Looking for a quick way to assess your daily dose of "news-trition"? Watch for these ten red flags of junk science from the Food and Nutrition Alliance (FANSA):

1. Recommendations that promise a quick fix
2. Dire warnings of danger from a single product or regimen
3. Claims that sound too good to be true
4. Simplistic conclusions drawn from a complex study
5. Recommendations based on a single study
6. Dramatic statements that are refuted by reputable scientific organizations
7. Lists of "good" and "bad" foods
8. Recommendations made to help sell a product
9. Recommendations based on studies published without peer review
10. Recommendations from studies that ignore differences among individuals or groups

If you've been taken in by a junk science claim:

- *Check it out with a reliable source:* a registered dietitian, your public health department, or your county Cooperative Extension office.
- *Report a statement, product, or service that appears fraudulent:* to the postal service if it came through the mail; to the Food and Drug Administration (your regional FDA office) if it's about a dietary supplement; and to the Federal Trade Commission (1-877-FTC-HELP) if it's an advertising claim.

November 30   Calories Out? Calories In!

Eat out often? If so, you may consume more calories than people who eat more meals at home. A U.S. Department of Agriculture study says that people who eat out often tend to weigh more.

Order smart with a healthful-eating mind-set.

- *Take the edge off your appetite.* Drink water before ordering.
- *Split an order.* You'll split the calories. Or consider the appetizer menu for your main dish.
- *Indulge often in:* clear soup, salad dressing on the side, grilled meat, steamed or roasted veggies.
- *Order less often:* creamy soup, salad with dressing, breaded meat or entrées with gravy, fried veggies.
- *Move the basket of tortilla chips or bread elsewhere.* A 3-cup chip basket may have 400 calories or more.
- *Watch dipping oil.* A slice of bread may soak up 3 to 4 teaspoons of olive oil (14 to 19 fat grams, or 126 to 171 calories), twice as much as a typical 1½ to 2 teaspoons of butter spread!
- *Give yourself a one-drink maximum.* Drinks add up: 100 calories for 5 ounces of dry wine, 150 calories for 12 ounces of beer, and 150 calories or more for a small mixed drink.
- *Order sorbet, fruit, or cappuccino for dessert.*

December 1   Prancing and Dancing

Holiday season seem too hectic for your usual fitness routine? That's no reason for a holiday from physical activity. Guidelines don't change. The 60 minutes of daily physical activity you need to keep fit may be the perfect antidote for relieving seasonal stress and weight gain.

Dovetail physical activity with seasonal festivities.

- *Use the mall's stairs, not the escalator*—at least until your feet hurt.
- *Enjoy active household tasks that make the season glitter:* decorating the house, polishing silver, kneading holiday bread dough, chopping firewood.

- *Decorate outdoors.* With kids, drape cranberry and popcorn chains on evergreens to feed the birds. For ornaments, roll pinecones in peanut butter and birdseed.
- *Put action in family gatherings.* Move away from the dinner table, put leftovers away (perhaps leave the dishes 'til later), and encourage everyone to join in active fun. Walk a nearby trail, go caroling, make a snowman, sled in the park, go snowshoeing, or play touch football, weather permitting.
- *Sneak in a fitness stop.* After running holiday errands, a 30-minute workout and a 10-minute sauna may feel great.

December 2   Stress-less Holiday

Are holiday expectations making you stressed? Are you tempted to eat your holiday cookies right away instead of saving them? Are seasonal time demands competing with your daily eating and exercise routine?

Here are some ways to cut holiday stress and keep control of your personal fitness:

- *Organize.* Plan ahead, keep to-do lists, combine errands. Save your holiday time and energy for what's fun and festive.
- *Say "no"*—to problems you can't resolve, to demands that exhaust you, to things you don't enjoy, to tasks that aren't yours, especially if your calendar is already full. You don't need to organize food for the office party if you're chairing a school fund-raiser!
- *Take care of you.* Eat smart, stay active, sleep enough. Staying fit gives you more energy and "cool" to deal with holiday stressors. Avoid pressures from others' expectations.
- *Expect setbacks; just move on.* Your dog's muddy paws *will* mess up your carpet just before party time. Weather *will* delay guests.
- *Accept your limitations.* You're wiser to do less better than do more badly. You don't have to make gingerbread ornaments just because you always have. You *can* host a crowd, but only if each guest brings a dish.
- *Do tough tasks first.* Once done, their stresses are off your mind!

December 3   Eat, Think, and Be Merry

Throwing a holiday party? If you plan to serve alcoholic drinks, host responsibly. Plan ahead so a cocktail, beer, or glass of wine can be part of the festivities—without putting a damper on your guests' fun and personal safety.

For the record, a healthy body can detoxify about one drink per hour; drinking coffee won't speed the process. What counts as a drink? A 12-ounce beer, a 5-ounce glass of wine, a 1½-ounce jigger of distilled spirits (bourbon, whiskey, rum). They all have roughly the same amount of alcohol, ½ ounce pure ethanol.

When you host a party now—or any time—with alcoholic drinks:

- *Downsize drinks.* "Supersizing" encourages excessive drinking. Use a 1-ounce, not a 1½-ounce, jigger.
- *Pair drinks with food.* Their flavors can complement each other. What's more, eating slows alcohol absorption.
- *Offer nonalcoholic options.* Serve no-alcohol wine or beer, sparkling water, or a festive punch, giving choices for everyone.
- *Ensure a safe way home.* Plan for designated drivers. Or be prepared to call a taxi.

December 4   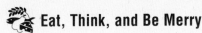 Shop, Wrap, Ship

Giving food gifts this season? Great idea—*if* they keep their peak quality and stay clean and safe en route. Give recipients a heads-up so your gift doesn't sit out too long.

Pack gifts in clean, well-protected containers. Pack perishables frozen or refrigerator cold, in an insulated cooler or heavy box with cold packs or dry ice. Mark "Perishable—Keep Refrigerated" and ship for overnight delivery.

Open any food gifts you receive immediately. Perishable foods don't stay safe or keep the best quality for long, even in the refrigerator. Some cured meats (hard salami, dry cured ham) don't need refrigeration. Perishables, including other meats and most hams, fish, and poultry, should be refrigerator cold on arrival. If not, toss; request a replacement or a refund.

Consider sending these healthful, holiday food gifts:

- *Fresh fruit.* Some mail-order houses specialize in shipping seasonal fruit.
- *Nuts and dried fruit.* Fill a fanciful bowl with your creative trail mix.
- *Spice and herbal teas.* Pack containers of loose tea or tea bags with colorful mugs.

December 5   ✒ Cook Savvy—Baker's Half Dozen

Ready to start your holiday baking? Baking experts advise using quality ingredients and measuring carefully. Use soft, not melted butter or margarine—unless the recipe says to melt. Preheat your oven. Use the suggested pan size. Follow doneness advice. Cool on a rack.

Experiment for nutrition. The results may differ from what you're used to.

- *For more fiber*

    Go 50-50. Use half white flour, half whole-wheat flour.

    Add fruit or nuts: dried berries, currants, apricots, apples, papaya, dried plums (prunes); and almonds, walnuts, pecans, pistachios, hazelnuts, peanuts. Try fresh pomegranate seeds!

- *For less fat and/or cholesterol*

    Substitute puréed fruit: Use applesauce, puréed dried plums, or mashed bananas for half the butter, margarine, or oil. (Great for bar and drop cookies)

    Try yogurt in place of sour cream in biscuit or muffin batter, or bread dough.

    Use egg whites in place of some (not all) whole eggs. Using only whites toughens baked goods.

- *For less added sugar*

    Reduce sugar by 25 to 33 percent, unless the recipe's already been adjusted. For good results, for each cup of flour, plan ½ cup sugar in cakes; 1 tablespoon sugar for muffins and quick breads; 1 teaspoon sugar for yeast breads.

December 6 'Tis the Season

Be jolly and enjoy party food! But with all the eating and drinking that goes with entertaining, how can you avoid what may seem inevitable—seasonal weight gain?

Extra weight comes from more than partying. Fewer daylight hours and busy social schedules often make fitness routines low priority. Cookies, candy, dips, and nog—many holiday foods are calorie laden with fat and sugar. And they're everywhere!

If you do add a pound or so of girth this holiday season, take steps to cut back in January. Otherwise the seasons add up: five Decembers, five pounds—consider how that adds up over a lifetime!

Before you party, decide how you'll keep party calories in control.

- *Count drink calories (see November 30).* They sneak up. Another option: Toast the season with sparkling water with a citrus twist.
- *Enjoy calorie-free party talk.* Socialize away from the party buffet.
- *Take off the hunger edge.* Before the party, nibble a low-calorie snack to quell your appetite at the buffet.
- *Take one trip to the table.* Survey it first. Then choose just what you really want. Just a little taste may satisfy your curiosity.
- *Dance if there's party music.* You'll burn calories!

December 7 It's a Cookie Exchange

Cookies, cookies, and more—an array of homemade cookies, served on a holiday plate, marks the season. But who's got time for all that baking? And how to resist indulging if you do bake?

Easy solution: just exchange! Invite a group of friends or coworkers to bring four dozen of their favorite cookies to swap, along with an empty container. Everyone goes home with a fabulous selection of four dozen cookies.

A few tips for healthier, tastier cookies:

- *Toast nuts (see March 8).* You get more flavor from less nuts.
- *Switch flour.* For a chewier, more fiber-rich bar, replace one-third all-purpose flour with oat flour. Grind your own oat flour from oats in your food processor.
- *Substitute dried fruit.* Use dried berries, cherries, raisins, or chopped dried apricots, plums, or apples in place of chocolate chips. A little crystallized ginger is good, too.
- *Skip the raw cookie dough.* Raw eggs in the dough carry a salmonella risk.

December 8   Pear-fect!

Want an easy taste adventure? Substitute ripe fresh or canned pears in any recipe that calls for apples: baked crisps, salads, even applesauce or baked apples. With a little citrus juice, fresh pears won't discolor.

Like apples, pears pack plenty of goodness. Peel on, a medium pear delivers just 100 calories and about 4 grams of dietary *fiber*. About half is cholesterol-lowering soluble fiber. They have some *vitamin C* and *potassium,* too. And their antioxidants, called catechins (a flavonoid), may help protect you from cancer.

Try pears in a spinach salad, a pear-cranberry smoothie, or on a turkey sandwich.

Pear Mincemeat Bars

¾ cup butter or margarine	½ teaspoon salt
¾ cup softened, packed brown sugar	½ teaspoon baking soda
1½ cups flour	2 Anjou pears, cored and chopped
1¼ cups quick rolled oats	1 cup prepared mincemeat
½ cup chopped walnuts	1 teaspoon lemon juice
	½ teaspoon grated lemon peel

Preheat oven to 375°F. Cream butter and sugar. Stir in flour, oats, walnuts, salt, and baking soda until mixture is crumbly. Press ⅔ of crumb mixture into a 9-by-13-by-2-inch pan. Combine pears, mincemeat, lemon juice, and peel; spread over crumb crust. Top with remaining crumb mixture; pat lightly. Bake 25 to 30 minutes or until crust is golden. Makes 48 bars.

Source: Pear Bureau Northwest

December 9   🍎 Hey, "Sugar"

Want to sweeten your pot with flavor, not calories or added sugars? Then experiment with sugar substitutes (intense sweeteners). You get sweet taste with just a tiny fraction of the calories—especially useful if you're managing your weight or diabetes. Intense sweeteners aren't carbohydrates, so they won't promote tooth decay either.

Check the supermarket shelf. You'll five FDA-approved types: (1) aspartame, made of amino acids. (*Note:* Skip this one if you have the rare genetic disorder, phenylketonuria.); (2) saccharin, made from a grape substance, no longer government-listed as a possible carcinogen; (3) acesulfame potassium; (4) sucralose; and (5) tagatose.

These sweeteners have different cooking qualities than sugar. You'll need to experiment!

- *Check for sugar equivalents and cooking advice.* They're printed on the label.
- *Go easy, because the flavor's so intense.* A little goes a long way in your smoothie, cereal, a tart fruit sauce, or any recipe.
- *Choose the right sweetener for heating.* Saccharin, acesulfame potassium, and sucralose stay sweet when heated. Aspartame doesn't.

December 10   🍴 Tradition, Tradition

Holiday breads, turkey with all the fixins', Grandma's veggie casserole bubbling in the oven: What foods conjure up your own family memories?

The family table is more than a place to eat together. Family food traditions bind families together, especially during the holiday season.

As part of your holiday celebrations, honor family food traditions.

- *Start recording your own parents' recipes.* Serve them often.
- *Create a family food history.* Invite your extended family to bring recipes from parents and grandparents. Compile them in a family cookbook. Great holiday gift!

- *Serve family dishes at your holiday table.* Invite your relatives to bring family dishes and their stories to share around the table.
- *Set the table with family treasures:* Grandma's dishes, Dad's carving set, children's table decorations, even family pictures.

December 11   Appe-teasers

Chips with sour cream dip, fried eggrolls or chicken wings, mayonnaise-based spreads with crackers—ever notice how these high-fat higher-calorie foods appear at nearly every holiday party? If you're hosting this season—or if you're bringing party food—set a new standard. Serve heart-healthy fare. Invite guests to bring a dish and do the same. (Even ask them to share their recipes.)

Start with these easy party ideas:

- *Make calcium-rich, yogurt-cheese party dip.* Drain gelatin-free, low-fat yogurt in a yogurt strainer or a paper coffee filter set over a bowl. Cover and refrigerate for 2 to 24 hours, to drain to desired consistency. Flavor with herbs, or blue cheese and apple, or salmon and green onion.
- *Bake low-fat "chips."* Cut wonton wrappers into wedges, spritz with vegetable oil spray, and dust with chopped herbs (oregano, rosemary) or garlic or chili powder. Bake at 350°F for 10 to 15 minutes, until crisp. Serve with fruit chutney or salsa.
- *Serve a red-and-green veggie platter.* Make guacamole with crunchy red pomegranate seeds, fresh cilantro, and lime juice. Serve with raw veggies: red bell pepper and grape tomatoes, and green beans, broccoli, celery, and zucchini spears. *Tip:* To brighten their color, microwave veggies (not tomatoes or celery) for 60 seconds or less, then plunge in cold water.
- *Serve a rainbow of fruit:* berries, kiwi, apple and pear slices, starfruit.

December 12   🛒 Just a Cup of Herbal Tea

Hot herbal tea on a chilly December day—sounds good! Ginger citrus tea, tension-relief herbal tea, peppermint tea all sound healthful. But are herbal teas any better for you than traditional teas?

Green, black, or oolong—tea appears to have health-promoting benefits. However, the health benefits of herbal teas haven't been studied; neither their benefits nor safety is really known. Some may interfere with medication. Be aware, too, that while many herbal teas are really tea-herb blends (see June 4), other herbal teas aren't really tea, but infusions of other plant parts.

Caution: A few herbs used to make "tea" may be harmful, especially in large amounts. Among them, comfrey may cause liver damage; lobelia, breathing problems; and woodruff, bleeding, since it's an anticoagulant. Chamomile is known to cause allergic reactions.

If you'd love to relax with a cup of herbal tea this weekend:

- *Buy a major brand of herbal tea.* It's likely safe to drink.
- *If you're taking medication, ask your doctor first.*
- *Add a cinnamon stick, ginger, peppermint, or rosemary as you infuse regular tea.* They, too, may have antioxidant power.

December 13   🔪 Through Thick or Thin

Love the creamy thickness of chowder? The velvety smoothness of vegetable bisque? The heartiness of harvest stew? The full body of these dishes often comes from heavy cream, a flour-butter roux, or egg yolks—adding calories, fat, and cholesterol, too.

Try these healthful culinary tricks to get you through the thick or thin of soup, stew, or chili:

- *To thicken, stir in*

    Mashed potatoes, sweet potatoes, squash

    Puréed beans, any kind

    Tomato paste

Bread cubes or crumbs

Leftover puréed veggies, rice, or pasta

- *To thin, stir in*

Fat-free or low-sodium broth

Liquid from cooking vegetables

Tomato juice

Fruit juice

Tuna Chowder

1 10¾-ounces can low-sodium chicken broth	½ cup chopped celery
1 cup diced potatoes	½ cup frozen corn
1 pound yellow fin tuna steaks, skinned and cubed	½ teaspoon dried basil
	¼ teaspoon dried thyme
½ cup chopped onion	½ cup low-fat milk
½ cup chopped carrots	1 tablespoon chopped parsley

In a large saucepan, mix broth with 1 can of water. Add potatoes and simmer 10 to 15 minutes until tender. Remove cooked potatoes from broth, reserving liquid. Purée cooked potatoes with ¼ cup broth. Add tuna, vegetables, seasonings, and puréed potatoes to remaining broth in saucepan. Simmer 8 to 10 minutes until fish flakes easily. Stir in milk and heat to serving temperature without boiling. Sprinkle with parsley just before serving. Makes 4 servings.
Source: National Fisheries Institute

December 14   Season of Giving

Just eleven more days until Christmas! Feeling time-pressed to finish your shopping? Then consider gifts to help others and yourself stay fit. What would encourage the people on your list to get 60 minutes of moderate physical activity every day?

Here are some ideas:

- *A fitness gift certificate.* Consider: fitness club membership, sports equipment store, community fitness class. (Wrap up a certificate for yourself, too!)
- *Active "toys"*

  For kids, in-line or ice skates, balls, bicycle, sled

For teens and adults, exercise gadget (heart-rate monitor, pedo-meter), jazzy water bottle, gym equipment, exercise videos

For pets (and you), a new toy or walking leash

For everyone, safety equipment (helmets, reflectors for clothing)

- *A winter family adventure.* Rent snowshoes or cross-country skis to enjoy in a nearby park. Or give the whole family just one big gift: a ski trip or a getaway for warm-weather activity.
- *Time.* By yourself or as a family, share time with someone else this season. Volunteer at a homeless shelter or a retirement center. Shovel snow for elderly neighbors, take out their garbage cans, run their errands. Help collect toys for needy kids.

December 15   Use Your Nog-gin

Does eggnog add seasonal flavor to holiday parties? Does hot buttered rum warm you up on cold December nights? Then enjoy. But before a few sips become a few cups, consider this: True eggnog has 340 calories (from sweeteners and fat) per cup. From egg yolks and full-fat milk, much of its 20 fat grams per cup is saturated. Mix in a 1½-ounce jigger of brandy or rum, and calories soar to 440—per cup!

For hot buttered rum, check the recipe! Its belly-warming flavor and calories come from the butter, brown and confectioner's sugar, rum, and sometimes ice cream.

Enjoy healthier versions of holiday beverages in place of dessert.

- *For eggnog*

   Buy lower-fat versions or soy eggnog. They have dramatically fewer calories, fat, and saturated fat.

   Buy the small carton—to ease temptation for more.

   Lighten up! Mix any store-bought eggnog with evaporated fat-free milk.

   Make over homemade eggnog recipes. Use evaporated fat-free milk instead of cream; for safety's sake, use pasteurized egg substitute in place of egg yolks.

- *For hot buttered rum:* Substitute tub margarine (less saturated fat and no cholesterol) for butter; reduce sugar; reduce alcohol— ½ to 1 teaspoon rum extract for 2 tablespoons rum; replace ice cream with frozen yogurt.
- *Mull cider* with a cinnamon stick instead of making hot buttered rum!

December 16 🩺 Tired Blood?

Ever said tired blood is why you felt so tired? Maybe you simply need more sleep. Or maybe you really *are* anemic.

Tired blood actually is a good way to define anemia. With anemia, blood cells can't carry as much oxygen to blood cells to make energy because the red blood cells are smaller or there are fewer of them. Less oxygen to cells can lead to fatigue, mild depression, poor concentration, and higher risk for infection.

Anemia has several causes: some nutritional, some not. Nutritional anemias may result from:

- *Not enough iron,* especially among children, teenage girls, and women of childbearing age. Iron in blood helps carry oxygen. (Menstrual loss and pregnancy increase iron need.)
- *Not enough folate,* but since most grain products are folic acid-fortified, that's less of a problem today.
- *Not enough vitamin B_{12}* can happen if you don't have enough "instrinsic factor" (a stomach chemical) for vitamin B_{12} absorption. Strict vegetarians (no animal sources of food) don't get enough vitamin B_{12} either.

If you think you have anemia:

- *Call for a physical exam*—for a proper diagnosis and to rule out other health problems.
- *Consume foods with iron.* (See February 28.) Take a supplement if needed.
- *Eat plenty of fruits, vegetables, and grain products*—all sources of folate.

December 17   Eggs—Another Option

Buying eggs isn't as easy as it used to be. The options aren't just medium, large, and jumbo. What should you buy?

Brown (versus white), organic, fertile, or free-range eggs: there are no nutritional advantages. For a single egg, each has about 10 percent of your day's *protein* need. Eggs supply *vitamins A, D,* and *B$_{12}$,* as well as *lutein* and *zeaxanthin;* and about 215 grams of cholesterol and 5 fat grams in a large egg.

Other options if they match your health needs:

- *Cholesterol-free liquid eggs (egg substitutes):* ¼ cup equals 1 whole egg. Sold in cartons, they're made from egg whites. (Yolks contain the cholesterol.)
- *Nutrient-modified shell eggs:* some with more heart-healthy omega-3 fatty acids, some with less cholesterol. Read the Nutrition Facts.

Watching your cholesterol? Try egg substitutes in holiday desserts.

Berry Silken Tofu Cheese Cake

¼ cup graham cracker crumbs (4 2½-inch squares)
¾ cup egg substitute (equivalent to 3 whole eggs)
10½ ounces silken firm tofu, drained and cubed

½ cup sugar
1 tablespoon lemon juice
1 teaspoon vanilla extract
1 cup nonfat ricotta cheese
1 cup berries or other fruit

Preheat oven to 325°F. Spray bottom of an 8-inch springform pan or pie pan with vegetable cooking spray. Evenly spread graham cracker crumbs on bottom of pan. Blend remaining ingredients (except berries) in food processor until smooth. Pour into pan, bake 35 to 40 minutes. Remove from oven, cool 15 minutes at room temperature. Refrigerate. Cut into 8 slices. Top with berries. Makes 8 servings.

Source: United Soybean Board

December 18   Wal-Nuts to You!

Today's nutrition advice is getting nutty! Eating a small handful of walnuts (eight to eleven nuts) or other nuts is good for you.

Because the *unsaturated fatty acids* in nuts don't raise cholesterol levels, nuts are heart-healthy. What's more, walnuts are an excellent source of *omega-3 fatty acids* that help keep blood vessels from clogging and help prevent arteries from hardening. All nuts are good sources of *protein, some minerals,* and *flavonoids* that can help fight cancer and heart disease, too.

Add a walnut accent.

- *To soup:* chopped walnuts on pumpkin or potato soup, corn or fish chowder
- *Over fish:* finely chopped walnuts on any baked or broiled finfish
- *In salads, wraps, and pasta:* toasted chopped walnuts mixed in (see March 8)
- *In batter:* chopped walnuts mixed in pancake, waffle, and muffin batter

Sunrise Power Blend

1½ cups strawberries, halved	¼ cup nonfat dry milk (optional)
2 ripe peaches,* pitted and quartered, or an additional cup of strawberry halves	3 tablespoons wheat bran or oat bran (optional)
1 cup fat-free yogurt	2 tablespoons honey
	¼ cup (1 ounce) chopped walnuts

Put all ingredients in a blender, and blend until smooth and frothy. Makes 2 (10-ounce) servings.

Source: Walnut Marketing Board

*Canned peaches may be substituted.

December 19   Solutions, Not Excuses

"It's snowing." "The dog ate my shoes." "My walking partner moved." Dump the barriers to active living. Focus on solutions instead!

- *"No time."* Fit active living "in between"; even 10 minutes here and there make a difference. Try for 60 minutes daily.
- *"Sweating ruins my hair."* Enjoy rigorous activity after work or on weekends when you can "let your hair down."
- *"Too tired."* Moving more just may boost your energy and release tension.

- *"Too old to start."* You're never too old! Do whatever matches your skill and interest. Work up from slow walking to moderate walking to brisk walking.
- *"Not athletic."* That's okay. Do what "moves" you: an active hobby, home repairs, dog walking.
- *"No place to exercise nearby."* You can walk nearly anywhere: around the parking lot, down the corridor, in a park. Or march in place, swinging your arms, while you watch your favorite TV show.
- *"Healthy and trim without it!"* Remember: Being trim or having a BMI of 18.5 to 25 isn't necessarily being fit. Regular physical activity lowers risk for many health problems.

Any of these excuses sound familiar? If not, jot down your excuses and commit to finding a solution for each!

December 20 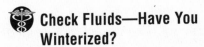 Check Fluids—Have You Winterized?

As you perspire in the summer heat, drinking to quench your thirst is usually automatic. Now that it's winter, remember that cold weather can be risky for dehydration, too, and not just for those who sweat from rigorous outdoor winter activities.

Water is part of your body's cooling system. In very cold weather, as in hot, your body uses water to maintain its normal temperature. Heated, recirculated indoor air dries moisture from your skin. Dry winter air also promotes dehydration. And bundled in layers of clothes, you may perspire a lot, even outside in the cold.

To keep your fluid levels normal any time of year:

- *Take regular water breaks.* Make that a habit at home, work, or play.
- *Keep bottled water handy*—at your desk, in your car (if it won't freeze), when you work out, in your briefcase.
- *Drink before, during, and after rigorous activity.* Shoveling snow? Skiing or winter hiking? Carry bottled water along.

December 21   ✇ A Little Light on a SAD Subject

Winter solstice—the shortest day in a season of long, dark nights. Many people suffer from the "winter blues" or its more severe form, Seasonal Affective Disorder (SAD). According to the National Mental Health Association, an estimated 25 percent of the population suffers from mild winter SAD, and about 5 percent, from its more severe form. SAD can affect anyone. The risk is highest for young people and women.

Common symptoms include depression, sadness, or moodiness; changes in sleep and eating habits; cravings for sugar or starchy foods; increased appetite, followed by weight gain; low energy and fatigue. SAD sufferers can't easily adjust their daily biological clock to shifts in sunlight patterns.

The reasons are not fully understood. But melatonin, a sleep-related hormone also linked to depression, may be a factor. The body produces more melatonin during short, dark days.

Make the winter solstice a time to get help for SAD.

- *Seek a physician's help first*—light therapy or medication for severe cases.
- *Physical activity helps relieve depression*—especially walking or other outdoor daytime activities.
- *Spend time outdoors.* Or arrange your indoor space to bring more sunlight in.

December 22   ✇ Chilled Out? Warm Up!

Do you need to eat more to keep warm? That's a tempting rationalization. But if your daily routine doesn't change, you don't need more calories. True, your body uses energy to stay warm. But you burn extra calories only if your body temperature drops enough to make you shiver.

That said, can food or drink take your chill away?

What works: Mom knew: a hot cup of cocoa, mulled cider, or a hearty bowl of chowder or chili. In fact, any hot food helps warm you from the inside out. And eating itself has a "heat-making" effect, as metabolism speeds up from energy released during digestion. That may be why your brain signals hunger when your body temperature drops.

What doesn't: Brandy or other alcoholic drinks tend to increase the body's heat loss, which makes you more susceptible to cold.

Stay warm this winter.

- *Outdoors, keep your water bottle inside your parka.* Drinking icy water chills your stomach and your whole body.
- *Carry a snack for winter activity.* If you're chilled, dried fruit or granola cookies may stoke your furnace.
- *Enjoy warm drinks:* simmered cranberry-apple juice with a cinnamon stick, or hot cocoa topped with a small scoop of praline frozen yogurt. (See January 21.)

December 23   Better Angle

Positioned comfortably by the TV this wintry evening? Americans, on average, watch nearly four hours of television daily—potentially a lot of sitting time. Yet we all know, fitting more movement into leisure time offers more long-term health benefits.

Get more from your TV time today.

- *Take a commercial action break!* You've got 10 to 12 minutes during a 30-minute network show to get up and do a quick household chore.
- *Watch a show that "moves" you.* Work out with a cable TV exercise program or dance to a televised concert.
- *Dust off the exercise bike, put it by the TV.* Watching the news while you cycle puts a more positive spin on the day's events.

December 24   'Twas the Night Before . . .

According to tradition, Saint Nicholas was the first to fill stockings—with gold coins to ensure happy marriages for three noble sisters who lost their mother. Today food and trinkets turn empty stockings into festive gift bags. Rather than the usual candy canes, chocolates, and small toys, why not stuff children's socks with health-focused goodies?

Fill stockings for those great girls and boys—adults, too—with:

- *Fresh fruit:* tangerines, oranges, apples, or pears
- *Dried fruit and nuts:* little packets of dried cranberries, blueberries, cherries, or raisins; almonds, pistachios, pecans, walnuts, or sunflower seeds
- *Kitchen stuff:* child's apron, measuring spoons, mini baking pans, potholders, or child's cookbook
- *Action stuff:* jump rope, Smurf ball, sweatband, fun gym socks, or a single-use camera (Let kids capture family memories.)

December 25 Healthy Holiday—All about You

No matter how—or why—you may celebrate, it's Christmas Day. As you enjoy family and friends, make healthful choices together that match your individual lifestyles.

For the best gift of the season—good health.

- *Be realistic.* Stick with your small steps to eat smart and move more. Enjoy vegetables served at dinner. Serve yourself a reasonable portion of turkey or meat (or dessert). Go light with gravy.
- *Be adventurous.* Try new foods today if your host prepared or a guest brought something you've never tasted. You'll expand your tastes to enjoy more food variety.
- *Be flexible.* No need to worry if you indulged your taste buds today. Make it up in the next few days with light meals and mall walking as you hit the postholiday sales.
- *Be sensible.* Enjoy the holiday spread, just push away from the table when you're done. Skip everyday dips and chips so you have room for that special, perhaps traditional, once-a-year dessert.
- *Be active.* After dinner enjoy a family Christmas Day walk. Play Ping-Pong. Dance together.

December 26   🥄 Passport to Health—Eating with African American Flavor

Keep the holiday spirit. Today starts Kwaanza, a weeklong African American commemoration of renewal, patterned after the African harvest celebration. Its name comes from the Kiswahili word *ku-anza,* meaning "to begin."

Symbols of Kwaanza have universal meaning. This first day honors *umoja,* or unity, among family as well as the community, the nation, and the world African community. Whatever your ethnic background, celebrating Kwaanza with traditional African American fare offers time to relax and renew the joys of the family table.

Consider preparing foods with African American roots: black-eyed peas and rice, okra and stewed tomatoes, gumbo, sweet potato pudding, cooked collards or turnip greens, among others.

Sweet Potato Fritters

1 pound sweet potatoes, peeled and coarsely shredded
3 large eggs
¼ cup chopped green onions
3 tablespoons all-purpose flour
½ teaspoon salt
¼ teaspoon ground mace
¼ cup vegetable oil

Wrap sweet potatoes in a clean dish towel; wring to remove excess moisture. In bowl, combine sweet potatoes with remaining ingredients except oil; blend well. Heat oil in large nonstick skillet over medium-high heat. Spoon heaping tablespoonfuls of batter into skillet, flattening with back of spoon. Cook until golden on both sides, turning after about 4 minutes. Remove from pan; place on paper towels to drain. Repeat with remaining batter. Serve with Coulis (recipe follows). Makes 6 servings.

Pear Coulis: In bowl, combine 2 chopped ripe pears, ¼ cup raisins, ½ cup orange marmalade, and 1 tablespoon finely chopped crystallized ginger.

North Carolina Sweet Potato Commission

December 27   🍎 It's Date Night

Dates add a flavorful complement to romantic dinners for two. Enjoy this peak season for this nutritious and sweetest of fruits.

Seventy-percent sugar by weight, dates have a candylike sweetness. Unlike other fruits, dates have essentially no vitamin C. Yet even five or six dates deliver *fiber* and *potassium,* and no fat.

Sweeten your cooking with dates.

- *Slivered and tossed in salads*—with Bibb lettuce or baby spinach, mandarin oranges, and toasted pecans
- *Chopped and mixed in pilaf, couscous, curries, or stir-fries*—in fact, in any recipe that calls for raisins
- *In desserts*—for an easy parfait, layer pineapple, raspberries, yogurt, banana, and dates; top with almonds. Add chopped dates to cookie, brownie, or quick bread dough.

December 28   Weight Loss? Think Again

Gained weight this season? Before you're lured by January promotions that advertise "fat-melting," "appetite-suppressing," "metabolism-boosting" weight-loss aids, get your guard up! Even if they foster short-term results, they're likely ineffective in the long run.

First, two gimmicks: Electric muscle stimulators don't really work your muscles, so you don't burn calories. Rubber belts and nylon clothes that make you sweat promote water loss, not fat loss.

About a few weight-loss supplements: Products with ephedra may suppress appetite and slightly boost metabolism; however, the U.S. Food and Drug Administration notes serious adverse effects (high blood pressure, rapid heartbeat, stroke, to name a few), especially when taken with caffeine. Taking guarana to make ephedra more potent makes it potentially more harmful. Conjugated linoleic acid (CLA) probably won't promote weight loss, but it probably won't hurt you either. Chitosan may reduce fat absorption (and fat-soluble vitamins), but its effectiveness and long-term safety isn't known. And chromium, which helps regulate insulin, probably won't promote weight loss or improve muscle mass much, if at all; it also can be toxic in high doses.

If a weight-loss product sounds too remarkable, it probably is! The Federal Trade Commission reports that 55 percent of weight-loss ads make misleading or false claims.

Before you buy:

- *Check with a registered dietitian.* Find a local expert through www.eatright.org.
- *Talk to your doctor,* especially if you take other medications.

December 29   Boost Your "Burn"

You know the basics: a pound of body fat equals 3,500 calories. To trim down, eat fewer calories, burn more, or do both. You get out of it what you put into it. So, the more often you're physically active, the longer you do it, and the harder you move, the more calories you burn. Just showing up for exercise or socializing your way through its motions won't burn much.

Calories Burned for Every 5 Minutes	120-Pound Person	170-Pound Person
Aerobic dancing	28	38
Bicycling (<10 mph)	18	26
Calisthenics	21	29
Cross country skiing	37	51
Jogging	32	45
Skating	32	45
Swimming, leisure	28	38
Walking, brisk	18	26
Driving	7	13
Sitting at the TV	4	6

To boost your burn:

- *Pump it up.* Use hand weights when you walk. Wave your arms as you dance.
- *Just add five.* Five more minutes of physical activity daily add up to more than 30 minutes a week. So, if you burn 18 calories for every 5 minutes of brisk walking, that's 126 calories a week more—if you just add 5!
- *Switch gears.* Simply walking more and sitting less makes a big difference. Take the stairs, do housework, shovel snow.

December 30 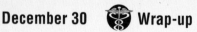 Wrap-up

Over this past year, you've explored the positives: what you can eat, not what you can't, for health. You've "tasted" what's known so far about the wide variety of health-promoting foods. And you've learned how many of those foods may protect you from heart disease and cancer.

This chart sums up some reasons why food variety helps promote your health!

	Foods with Potential Benefits	What May Give Those Benefits
For Heart Health	Beans, peas, barley	Soluble fiber, saponins
	Soybeans, other soy-based foods (not oil)	Soy protein, isoflavones, saponins, plant sterols, maybe fiber
	Oats, flaxseed (ground)	Soluble fiber, lignan
	Citrus fruit	Flavonoids, ferulic acid, caffeic acid
	Salmon, albacore tuna, sardines, mackerel, eggs with omega-3s	Omega-3 fatty acids
	Onions, scallions, shallots, garlic, leeks	Allyl sulfides
	Red grapes, purple grape juice, red wine	Resveratrol, ellagic acid
	Vegetables	Plant sterols, ferulic acid, antioxidant vitamins, fiber
	Nuts (almonds, walnuts, pecans, hazelnuts, others)	Phytic acid, arginine, plant sterols
	Tea (green or black)	Catechins
	Yogurt, buttermilk with live cultures	Probiotics
	Some cholesterol-lowering spreads	Plant stanol and sterol esters
For Cancer Protection	Vegetables, fruits	Antioxidant vitamins, phyto-nutrients* (allyl sulfides, anthocyanins, catechins, ellagic acid, isoflavones, lignan, limonoids, lutein, lycopene, saponins, sulphoraphane, fiber) *Different foods supply different phytonutrients.

Foods with Potential Benefits	What May Give Those Benefits
Beef, dairy foods, lamb	Conjugated linoleic acid
Yogurt, buttermilk with live cultures	Probiotics
Low-fat foods	Low in total fat and saturated fat
Tea (green or black)	Catechins
Flaxseed (ground)	Lignans, fiber
Soybeans	Isoflavones (genistein)

Source: R. L. Duyff, *American Dietetic Association Complete Food and Nutrition Guide* (New York: John Wiley & Sons, 2002).

With these benefits in mind:

- *Add one more fruit and vegetable serving,* or *whole-grain food* to your food choices today!
- *Turn back.* Read again about these foods.

December 31   Time to Reflect, Look Ahead, Celebrate

When the clock strikes midnight, how will you ring in the New Year? Will you reflect back on how you achieved your fitness goals over the past twelve months? Will you rethink and update next year's approach to healthful eating and active living?

The smart approach: Do both. Review what you've learned this past year to strategize for the coming one.

Celebrate with healthful New Year food folklore:

- *Enjoy a Cuban tradition:* twelve grapes eaten as the clock strikes midnight with one wish for each month of the year (Make twelve promises for fitness!)
- *Add Southern tradition to your midnight buffet:* Hoppin' John

(black-eyed peas cooked with ham and seasonings, and served with cooked rice) as a symbol of good luck.
- *Try a fishy Polish and German tradition:* herring at midnight for good luck.

Wishing you a Happy, Healthy New Year!